more simpler times

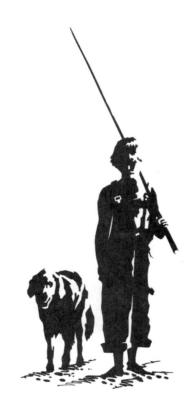

Tales of a Southern Boy

Charles D. "Pedro" Williams, MD

Illustrations by Marc L. Thomas
Cover Photo by Scott Holstein

ISBN 978-0-615-22492-3

Printed in the United States of America.

Published by Rowland Publishing, Inc.
1932 Miccosukee Road, Tallahassee, Florida 32308

Printed by Rose Printing Company, Inc.
2503 Jackson Bluff Road, Tallahassee, Florida 32314

Distributed by Capital Medical Society Foundation
1204 Miccosukee Road, Tallahassee, Florida 32308

First Edition – 2008

ACKNOWLEDGEMENTS

I'd like to thank my wife, Pat, for her support and encouragement while writing these stories. She was always by my side and she laughed when I laughed and cried when I cried.

A special thanks goes to my Grandma for encouraging me to go off to college and git a "dilemma," which I now have hanging on my wall.

Pedro once again gives a heap of thanks to Moultrie, Georgia — a town that gave love, direction, discipline, guidance, and support. A town that was his family and a town that helped him git raised rite.

Pedro appreciates the Capital Medical Society, the Florida Radiological Society, and the Florida Medical Association for their encouragement to write about his upbringing and also for providing a forum in their newsletters.

I sincerely appreciate the support and wisdom that Dr. Charles Moore, editor of the FMA Bulletin, gave over the many years. Dr. Moore knew a lot of big words and tried to teach me some. I also knew a few big words, such as "watermelon" and "refrigerator." A lot of what I learned was from my own backyard.

A special thanks goes to Nancy Ellison for always typing thangs rite.

I'd also like to mention the folks at Rowland Publishing: Brian Rowland for taking on the work, Shannon Grooters for overseeing the project to completion, Beth Nabi for her great designin' skills, Marc Thomas for his dead-on illustrations, and Scott Holstein for his purty pictures.

It is hoped that the proceeds from these stories will contribute in some small way to the We Care Program to provide medical care to those who cannot afford it.

Sincere thanks is given to the Capital Medical Society Foundation and Sunbelt Medical Publishers for the success of the first book, *Simpler Times*, which had five published editions.

On the Cover: Charles William "Will" Dailey, age nine, grandson of Charles D. Williams and his wife, Pat, and son of Charlie and Sharon Dailey. Will was photographed at the author's homesite in Tallahassee with Annie, who belongs to Will's first cousins, Dillon and Chase Andrews.

INTRODUCTION

More Simpler Times is a sequel to Dr. Williams' first book, Simpler Times, and is a collection of stories about growing up in South Georgia in the 1940s during the time when life was less complicated — a time when people had to make over, make do, or do without. Written through the eyes and innocence of "Pedro" (pronounced "Pee-dro"), Dr. Williams reflects on the wisdom and humor of his Grandma and her three boys — Millard, Dillard, and Willard.

Dr. Williams believes that laughter is the best medicine. It's a lesson the Tallahassee physician learned from his Georgia Grandma who weathered the trials of sharecropping with grace and style — dispensing slogans like, "The main thang is to keep the main thang the main thang."

It is hoped that these stories will warm and touch your heart and tickle your mind. By revealing the source of Dr. Williams' roots and background in the 1940s, may this stimulate some special memory from your past. We need to understand and appreciate where we came from so that we can recognize where we are. It is hoped that you laugh at these stories, laugh at yourself, and look back at your own Simpler Times with special memories and love for your kinfolks and family.

This book is a fundraiser for the We Care Program, which provides medical care for the indigent and is sponsored by Capital Medical Society Foundation. For more information about We Care, please call the Capital Medical Society at (850) 877-9018. Copies of Dr. Williams' book can be obtained by calling the same number or they can be purchased directly from the Tallahassee Memorial Hospital Gift Shop.

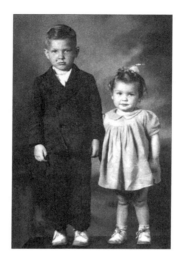

Pedro and sister, Mary Alice

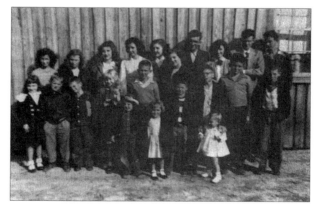

Grandma Williams' grandkids
Pedro (wearing glasses, third from right)

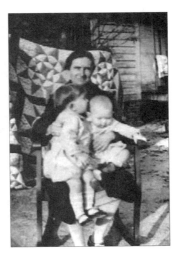

Grandma Williams with grand young'uns
One of grandma's quilts hanging behind her

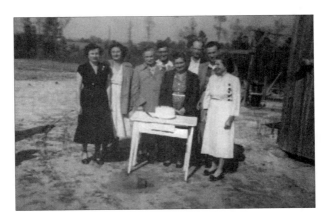

Grandma Williams (third from left) and her seven kids,
including sons Willard, Dillard, and Millard (back row, left to right)

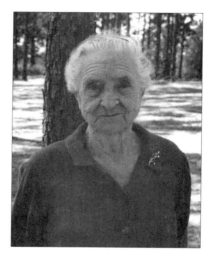

Pedro's grandma, Annie Caroline Williams
Feb. 13, 1892–Jan. 27, 1980

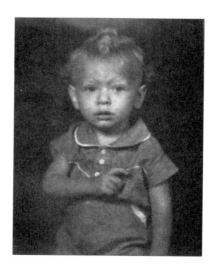

Charles D. "Pedro" Williams
Born March 24, 1940, in Colquitt County, Georgia

"PEDRO"

C harles D. Williams, MD, FACR, FAAP, was born at home in the country in Colquitt County on Cook Road near Jerusalem Church between Moultrie and Berlin, Georgia, on March 24, 1940. Grandma took it on herself to nickname him "Pedro." She was the same person who named her boys Millard, Dillard, and Willard. Pedro was born little and poor, but loud and proud.

With help from the good folks in Moultrie, Pedro went north to college and attended Mercer University in Macon, Georgia, receiving his AB in 1962. He then earned his medical degree from the Medical College of Georgia in 1966. He did his internship and residency in General Practice at the Medical Center of Central Georgia, finishing in 1968.

Dr. Williams served as a Captain in the United States Air Force Medical Corps at Homestead Air Force Base from 1968 to 1970. He went on from military duty to complete a residency in Diagnostic Radiology at Baylor College of Medicine in Houston, Texas, in 1973, serving as Chief Resident in 1972–73. Dr. Williams completed a fellowship in Pediatric Radiology at Shands Teaching Hospital, University of Florida College of Medicine, in 1973–74.

He is currently active in the private practice of radiology with Radiology Associates of Tallahassee. Dr. Williams has served as Vice President of the American College of Radiology and President of the Florida Radiological Society (FRS), and has served on the American College of Radiology Board of Chancellors. He also chaired the Commission of Human Resources for the American College of Radiology. Dr. Williams was the recipient of the FRS Gold Medal, the highest honor given to Florida radiologists. He was selected by *RT Image* as one of 2004's "most influential" among individuals, institutions, and organizations in radiology. Dr. Williams was also recognized in *Ladies' Home Journal* and *Redbook* for his work in medicine. He has always been active on the medical staff at Tallahassee Memorial Hospital, and served as Chief of Staff in 1986.

In spite of all his "edukashun," he never lost his sense of appreciation for his roots and his love for family. He and his wife, Pat, have six children and fourteen grandchildren. Spending time with the family is one of their greatest joys. They both love to garden and dig, as long as it is not for survival.

Contents

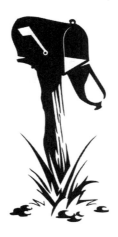

Precious Memories and Wrinkled Hands

I was sittin' on the back porch with my wife, Pat, reflectin' on our grand-kids and then remembered that a special gift of my childhood was havin' my Grandma and the special memories and lessons she left be-hind. She once told me that one day I would bundle up all my yesterdays and head for a tomorrow but it would be the memories of my yesterdays that would get me through my tomorrows.

Grandma has passed on but I'm so glad she passed my way. The only thangs she had to pass on to Pedro were her memories.

Grandma touched a part of my life that can only be handed down in stories. She used her stories to teach us about life. It didn't come from books on parenting. It had come from her mama who had learned it from her mama. It was not always what she said with her mouth but what I felt from her heart and saw in her eyes. For many of us, the old times were the best of times, or at least it seems that way.

Grandma and I spent time catchin' lightnin' bugs, making homemade ice cream in a hand-cranked churn, and spittin' watermelon seeds off the front porch, but my main most favorite memories were when we went walkin' and talkin'. She would reach down with her strong but wrinkled hands, which were like dried apples, and say, "Pedro, I want to spend some time with you. Let's go walkin'."

Back when Pedro was still wet behind the ears and littler'n most folks his age, Grandma and I walked down our long dirt road to get our mail from our rusty tin mailbox, which had some of our last name spelled rite. Some folks said that we lived so far back between Moultrie and Doerun that we got the Saturday night Grand Ole Opry on Tuesdays. They were teasin', I think. I do know that we got the Saturday paper on Tuesday. As we walked, Grandma said it was OK to be little but I might need to run twice as fast to keep up. She also said that no tree gits too tall that a short dog cain't tee tee on it and a person shuldn't git too big for their britches.

Another main most favorite time would be our walks through the garden. We walked past the corn fields as Grandma talked with a twinkle in her eyes and a joy in her heart. She could rip an ear of corn from the stalk, clean and strip the husk from each ear, and toss it in a basket. As we walked and Grandma talked, she said to watch out for snakes but most of the time they were more scareder of us than we were of them. I cudn't imagine anything that scared. She told Pedro to go off to college and git educated and git a dilemma and I did just that but it has taken me a long time to git over it.

Grandma said that she loved this dirt but she loved Pedro more. Diggin' helped her to git recharged. She told Pedro that if he ever found himself in a deep hole to stop diggin'.

One time, Willard gave her a new thermos. On one of our walks through the garden she threw the thermos under her arm as we headed out. I asked, "Grandma, what's a thermos?" She replied, "A magic jug. It keeps hot thangs hot and cold thangs cold." I said, "What you got in it?" She giggled and responded, "Hot chili and iced tea." I think she was pullin' my leg.

Another time on the way to the garden, we passed by the barn and the mule shed and Grandma asked, "Has that mule ever kicked you?" Pedro replied, "No, but he did kick one time right where I had been."

Even when communication became worldwide and instantaneous from way far off, nothing could beat goin' home and holdin' Grandma's hand and lookin' her in the eyes. She gave me such precious memories, a gift she gave unknowingly, or perhaps she did know. Maybe that's why she took the time. I had no idea how to thank her and never did have an idea. A government man once asked her if she had an ID and she replied, "About what?"

Recently, my grandson was visitin' and I took him for a short walk to the mailbox. I started tellin' him to wash behind his neck, to study hard in school, and to keep on the sunny side of life. As I was holdin' his hand, I felt a twinkle in my eye and looked down and noticed a few wrinkles in my hand. A chill set in my body and wetness set in my eyes. I then remembered that the memories Grandma left behind were the only thangs that her death didn't take away. I then turned to my grandson and said, "You're a special little man. Let's go for a long walk."

When the day ended, I leaned back in my rockin' chair, closed my eyes, and heard Grandma sing, "Precious memories, how they linger ... ." I must have fallen asleep. I think.

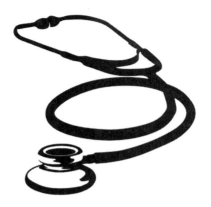

OLD-TIMEY DOCTORS
NEVER DIE

I was on the way to the hospital in my new truck, with my new phone, trying to act like a doctor when my mind drifted back to the doctors of Simpler Times. With Doctor's Day coming up, I wondered if we had truly made progress. It has been said that progress is trying to make things as good as they used to be.

Colquitt County in South Georgia, just like many other counties in North Florida, has had many outstanding, dedicated physicians over the past fifty years that have left their mark on many of the residents of these areas. There was a special trust for the medical community and there was a special bond between the doctor and patient just this side of kinship. So often, the doctors were paid in farm commodities in lieu of cash during the "hard years." Many of these doctors never made national prominence but they will live on in the hearts and minds of the local people. I could not possibly list or describe them all, but there were those that came into contact with Pedro's life that were typical of the many fine doctors during that era.

One of these special doctors was Dr. McGinty, who graduated from Emory and was headed to Miami to practice. On the way down, he spent the night in Moultrie and stayed from 1930 to his retirement in 1978. He brought Pedro into this world at Millard's shotgun house while Dillard and Willard sat out on the front porch and worried. Dillard tried to git comfortable and took off his shoes, scratched himself, wiped his nose, and turned to Willard and asked, "Do you mind if I smoke?" Later Dr. McGinty came out on the porch and told them Pedro had arrived and Willard said, "Praise the Lord."

Dr. McGinty did not know ever'thang, but he did git to know Pedro, and he knew Pedro's dog's name and Pedro's dog's best friend. He had a lifelong relationship with our family and he didn't have to write it down. He also knew we would eventually pay when we could and how we could. Millard paid him for Pedro's delivery with eggs and cream, and two weeks later delivered him a fresh ham.

Another one of these physicians was Dr. Gay, who arrived shortly after the outbreak of World War II in 1942 and was active in family practice for forty-six years. Dr. Gay told Pedro at age sixteen that if he wanted to be a doctor he needed to want to bad enough, and Pedro did. He gave us direction and strength when we were scared, and there were times he knew we were scared.

Another dedicated physician during Simpler Times was Dr. Paulk, who was the first accredited ophthalmologist in South Georgia. He first came to Moultrie in 1935 and practiced in Moultrie for forty years and specialized in eyes, ears, noses, and throats. Folks came all the way over from Bainbridge to see him. Dr. Paulk gave Pedro glasses, which kept the big boys from hittin' him and the girls from kissin' him. In 1945, he told Pedro that he was a good boy, and I never forgot it. I've remembered it clearly over the years and I believed him. It must have been so 'cause he said it and he was our doctor.

These doctors were limited in their diagnosis and treatment. They did not have machines that clicked and clunked and buzzed and could not inspect your innards from the outside but they gave us so much more. They gave us hope, comfort, and direction, and we knew that they were our friends and almost like kinfolks.

The rural towns are now going from payment with ham hocks to managed care and utilization management. Reimbursement has gotten too complicated to figure out. However, maybe today's doctors can still be advocates for their patients and hopefully still influence a few young people's lives along the way. An MBA is not needed for that.

These doctors touched folks' lives in many ways beyond the art of healing. They helped Pedro and other young folks to grow up, and they served as a role model for the community. They're still influencing many lives long after they are gone. Doctors like them still live on in the thoughts and memories of the Pedros of the world. Their influence still remains and will be appreciated for many years to come.

I have never felt like I fully repaid them and I don't remember thanking them. Maybe them knowing Pedro became a doctor was thanks enough. I hope.

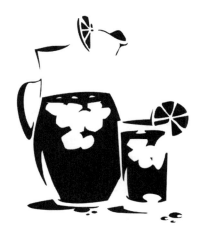

SOUTHERNERS
AIN'T IGNORANT

I was sitting at a table in the doctors' cafeteria with Dr. Yang, Dr. Patty, and Mr. Moore and we were talking about Southerners and how some folks think all Southerners are ignorant. This put me to thinking.

There's more to the South and Southerners than black-eyed peas, Moon Pies, kudzu, dinner on the ground, porch swings, prayer meetings, iced tea, wrestling, and fishing. There's a lot more. There's things like ugly dogs and boiled okra. Ugly dogs are happier in the South and boiled okra gives us our minimal daily requirements of fuzz and slime.

There's other things like straw hats, overalls, funeral home fans, and collard greens. Collards brought the races closer together.

Southerners meet and say, "How'zit goin'?" and "How'yah doin'?" These are greetings and not questions.

When Southerners congregate, the first type of conversation is weather, overnight comparison of thermometer readings, and the daily forecast. With the arrival of ever' new good ole boy, these comments will be rediscussed.

Then there's discussion of recent deaths, funerals, and ailments followed by crops, trucks, government, fishing, firearms, and whiskey. Whiskey is probably the most popular remedy that wudn't cure colds.

One pastime of Southerners seems to have gone by the wayside. That is snuff dippin'. I don't think it was the fear of cancer that stopped it, but that dippin' and spittin' didn't seem to go well with lovin'.

Another pastime is setting off firecrackers. One time, us young'uns went over to the county line and bought some fireworks for Christmas. We lighted our Roman candles and firecrackers and Grandma said, "You'd thought Jesus was a Cavalry officer." We then asked Grandma if she thought Jesus was a Southerner. She studied on it and said, "I don't think so, but he was good enough to have been one."

Some folks say us Southerners shoot anything that moves and put beer on our grits. Other folks say all us Southerners do is fish, tell stories, and read the Bible. That's not true. We also like to eat, and eating with family and friends was important. I'm not sure what our eatin' did to our bodies back then, but eating and fellowship brought our families closer together.

In South Georgia, us Southerners had to learn about makin' do. We had to make do, make over, or do without. It's about being good to your neighbor and neighbors helping neighbors and family helping family.

It seems that being Southern is a bunch of things. It's knowing where your people came from, how they got there, where they're buried, who married who or should've but didn't. It's the ability to be happy and thankful with simple things. Southerners try to keep things simple 'cause they're goin' to git complicated soon enough without us helping them along.

Being Southern is also the willingness to defend one's country and to fight for our freedom like many of 'em did in World War II. It's the ability to hold your head up, to keep your feet on the ground, to don't give up, to toughen up and hunker down. It's the ability to git your spirits energized with your hands in the soil. Being a Southerner is being proud of who you are and where you came from. Apparently, being a Southerner is also feeling comfortable with ending a sentence with a preposition.

One good thing about being a physician Southerner and having an MD back of your name is that it allows you to be yourself and talk the way you know how without folks thinking you're ignorant. That is — sometimes. That is — if you remain in the South.

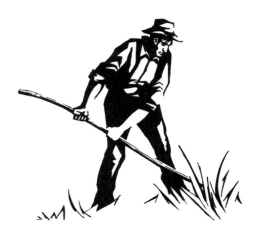

MY DAD

My dad is proud of me. I know he is. I saw it in his tears when I graduated from high school. He would have been just as proud of me if I had stayed in Moultrie and farmed. There are times I wished I had stayed and taken my place with the home folks. I know now it wouldn't be the same if I went back. Now Pedro has different shingles on his roof.

To me, Dad was a giant, but he was the tallest when he was on his knees. I saw a side of Daddy that most folks couldn't see. Six days out of seven he was up before dawn. He was a simple, hard-working country man trying to make a living, but he was at his best when his hands were in the soil. He had started from scratch and he kept scratchin'. One time, Dad told Pedro to watch where he scratched in public.

Dad was one of seven kids, including Millard, Dillard, and Willard. Grandpa died of the swine flu and we lost the farm. Grandma then moved on to somebody else's rundown farm to try sharecropping (tenant farming) with her seven kids. Grandma was gettin' the farm lookin' halfway decent when a friend from the Baptist church dropped by and said, "You, your young'uns, and the good Lord shore got this place lookin' good." Dad replied, "You should have seen it when the good Lord had it by Himself."

Dad tried to teach Pedro right from wrong. He didn't know big words or hard words, but he seemed to know what was important and what was not. He was smart enough to know when it was too wet to plow. He knew that you couldn't chase two rabbits at the same time and he knew you shouldn't step over a log that you couldn't see the other side of. He also knew that a person didn't have to hang from a tree to be a nut.

Dad taught Pedro a whole lot. He taught Pedro to wash up before supper, to eat his green beans, to thump watermelons, that BB guns could put your eyes out, and never to sass Mama. One time, Dad told Pedro not to speak when grown-ups were talkin'. Pedro replied, "I've tried that already and it don't work."

Dad didn't have no schoolin', but he did help Pedro to grow up. He raised Pedro right and he raised Pedro happy. Pedro got grown and found out that he was also raised poor, and found out he wudn't supposed to have been that happy. Dad also taught Pedro to stay between the ditches and out of other people's hen houses. One time, a neighbor had been messing around in someone else's hen house and he got shot. The doctor said that he had been shot between the hepatic flexure and the diaphragm, but Pedro said he had been shot between the hog pen and the barn. Grandma said that we were both right.

Dad hardly ever left Moultrie, but he did leave when he went to war to defend our country, when he went to see Hank Williams sing in Nashville, and when he went to see Pedro at Baylor in Houston. All big events. Even though he didn't travel much and even though he never got formally educated, he did learn to say "thank you" and "yes, ma'am" and "please." He also learned to give a dollar's worth of work for a dollar's worth of pay.

My dad never gave a great speech and never learned to conjugate a verb. However, I'm proud of my dad. I think he knows it. I think he saw it in my tears when he got sick. Father's Day is soon. I think I'll tell him.

Note: Dr. Williams' dad passed away shortly after this story was written.

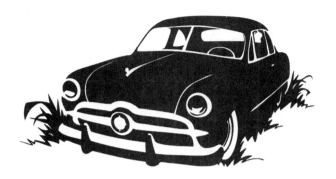

Those Sunday
Afternoon Drives

Sometimes I close my eyes and my mind starts wandering back to something in my past and I write it down so my young'uns can catch a glimpse of my heritage. It also gives me such pleasure when my thoughts go back to bygone days.

One of those special pleasures would be our Sunday afternoon drives in our 1949 Ford. Sometimes we would head out down any old dirt road. As Daddy talked, I believed the bumps in that dirt road prepared us for the bumps in our lives. Our values were better when our roads were worse. People did not worship their cars more than their kids, and drivers were more courteous. Once, Mama said if you don't know where you're going, any ole dirt road would do. The main idea was to git out of the house and see what was going on in the rest of our world. It was our way of catching up on the gossip, but Southerners called it spreading the truth.

Sometimes we'd set out from the southern end of Colquitt County and head to our kinfolks in the northern end of the county but we still considered them Southerners. We'd drop in on whoever happened to be home and not taking their own Sunday afternoon drives. We didn't call them beforehand 'cause we didn't have a phone. It didn't matter 'cause they didn't have a phone either.

We'd pile into that 1949 Ford, and that car brought us together and it kept us close together where we could talk and sing. Sometimes as we rode, we belted out songs and folks could hear us coming as we sang, "She'll be coming around the mountain when she comes and we'll kill the old red rooster when she comes." Sometimes with our singing, we would make Daddy as nervous as a long-tail cat in a room full of rocking chairs.

One time, Daddy said, "If you young'uns have to go tee tee, hold up two fingers." Pedro replied, "Daddy, how's that goin' to help?" Daddy then said that "a fool is just like other folks as long as he keeps his mouth shut."

Another time, Mama looked over into the back seat and noticed Pedro had the left shoe on the right foot and said, "Son, your shoes are on the wrong feet." Pedro looked up and said, "Mama, these are the only feet I got."

As we headed to visit our kinfolks we received much more. Daddy and Mama talked to us about life. I heard Mama tell Daddy that children were the riches of the poor. I then told Mama that I wanted to be somebody when I grew up but Mama said that I needed to be more specific.

As our eyes observed, our ears listened, and our minds processed the messages we received in the back seat of that 1949 Ford, the building blocks for a child's future were being laid. I listened very carefully 'cause I didn't want to make the wrong mistakes.

As I look back, I believe my life began to take shape in that 1949 Ford. All needs for nourishment and growth weren't physical. We were fed nourishment for our souls. I am the person I am today because of those Sunday afternoon drives. It was where hopes and dreams were shaped and the need for discipline was declared. We listened to each other and shared the reality of our lives. Character was developed in the back seat of that 1949 Ford. I wonder how I would have turned out if it had been a Chevy.

As I've gotten older I realize I learned a lot from those Sunday afternoon drives. As I've gotten older I've also learned that you miss your mama and daddy when they are gone from your life.

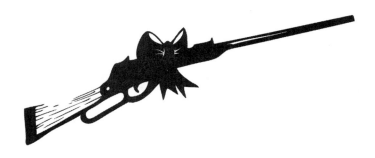

IS THERE REALLY
A SANTA CLAUS?

Christmas was Pedro's favorite time of the year. Mama would start
gettin' ready early by puttin' aside egg money, puttin' up preserves
for the market and takin' in sewing for some extra money. We thought we
were richer than we were, and in many ways we were.

Mama would bake extra pies, cakes, and puddin's, and kinfolks and
friends from all over would come to help celebrate the holidays and help
eat Mama's food. One time, Mama was serving some banana puddin' and
Pedro asked, "Will the dessert hurt me or is there enough to go around?"
Mama said that it was the Christmas season and there was plenty for
ever'body. Later she asked Emmett if he wanted a second helpin'. Emmett
told her that his mama said for him not to get a second helpin', but she
didn't know how small the first helpin' was gonna be.

Pedro always looked forward to the church play at Christmas. Pedro
usually got to play the donkey, 'cept the one time they used a real donkey.
At the Christmas play, ever'body practiced their parts. One time at the
play, Robert was going to be asked, "Who made you?" and he was supposed to answer, "God." The night arrived and the question was asked
three times. "Who made you?" Nobody responded until Thelma said,
"The little boy that God made is home with the chicken pox." The play
later concluded with the Off-Key Children's Gospel Singers.

In 1949, school let out for Christmas and Pedro and Emmett were riding the school bus home talking and thinking about Santa Claus. Emmett said that he had tried to be good and wanted a BB gun. Robert, who was listening to the coversation, said that last year on Christmas Eve he heard Santa Claus holler and mumble, "Dadgumit!" when he stumbled over his dog in the dark.

Pedro had gotten old enough and big enough and bright enough to know that if Santa Claus was going to bring him his favorite toys, he needed to pray real loud so Mama, Daddy, and Grandma could hear him. He also knew that it helped to turn down the pages in the Sears & Robuck catalog in the outhouse. Pedro wanted to believe in Santa Claus just like Emmett, who was younger.

Christmas morning arrived and there it was, the shiny new bicycle just like Pedro wanted. Also there was some fruit and a brand new Little Red Ryder BB gun with some Daisy BBs. Pedro couldn't wait to show Emmett and headed to Emmett's house. Upon arrival, Emmett looked over at Pedro barely able to speak and said, "Pedro, Santa Claus didn't come. Either I've been bad or he ran out of toys." Pedro could see the hurt in Emmett's eyes and hear the disappointment in Emmett's voice. Pedro, without thinking, replied, "Emmett, Santa did come. He thought you were spending the night with me and left your BB gun at my house. I was bringin' it to you."

Emmett grinned like a baked possum and was excited as a bug in a tater patch. Emmett hugged Pedro and Pedro hugged back. It was then at nine years old and there at that moment that Pedro once again learned there really was a Santa Claus.

On the way home on his new bike without his BB gun, Pedro kept thinkin', "Please, Mama, don't be mad," and she wasn't.

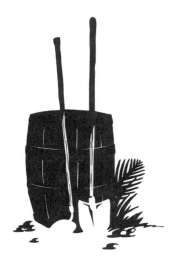

Ed's Gift to Pedro

When Uncle Ed went to meet his maker in 1979, word was sent to Pedro to come and git the hoe and shovel Ed promised him. They wudn't worth much on the open market but they were worth somethin' to Pedro. Ed knew that. He knew Pedro would remember.

Ed Murphy was Mama's half-brother. Mama said he was an Irishman. She said that you could always tell an Irishman, but you cudn't tell 'em very much. That's what Mama said.

In 1947, Mama told Pedro that because he had done good in school and that after he got treated for hookworms, he could go over to Uncle Ed's and Aunt Lourene's to spend a week pickin' blackberries. It was hard to wait but the day did come. Pedro and the dogs — Pete and Repete — would follow Ed around in the fields while he checked on things, chopped things, and pulled things. Pedro tried to help by carryin' the water jar.

One morning, we got an early start and headed to the blackberry patch way down the road just-a-walkin'. We stopped at the fork in the road to rest a spell and this rattle-trap car pulled up. The folks got out and we howdied and shook. They then asked Uncle Ed if it mattered which road they took to Pavo. Ed leaned on his hoe and studied on it and then replied, "No, it don't matter to us."

We then continued on to the blackberry patch and the dogs ran ahead. 'Bout then, there was a loud yep from Pete. Ed told Pedro to stay put and he grabbed the hoe and high-tailed it to the yepping. Ed hollered, "Rattlesnakes!" and started chopping as fast as he could with two snakes and one hoe. Things settled down and 'bout the time Pedro got there, Pete was deader than a doornail. Pedro started crying.

Elbert down the road heard the noise and came over to see what the racket was all about. Pedro, sobbing, looked at Elbert and said, "Pete's dead." Elbert then said that his grandmama died and he didn't even cry. Pedro wiped his eyes and said, "Yeah, but you ain't raised your grandmama from a puppy."

Me, Ed, and Repete started looking for a proper place for Pete to be laid to rest. We decided that over by the fence behind the smokehouse was pretty good since there were some wild roses growing over there. That way, Ed could keep check on him. We then laid Pete in the ground and started paying our proper respects. As Pedro leaned on Ed's shovel, Ed talked about dog heaven, how things like this hurt, how it was OK to cry, that we needed to talk about things, and other stuff I can't remember. Ed didn't have no Ph.D. and never heard of one. He didn't finish the fourth grade, but wished he had. On that day, Ed helped Pedro learn about death, hurt, therapy, support mechanisms, counseling, and bonding. Ed said that Pete had been faithful and that he had been a stomp-down good ole dog. Ed then gave one more holy piece of scripture for Pete and we sang, "Love lifted me, love lifted me, when nothing else could help, love lifted me." We picked up the hoe and shovel and headed back to the tool shed without saying a word. Upon entering the shed, Pedro asked, "Ed, when you die, can I have your hoe and shovel?" Ed smiled and said, "Yes, Pedro. Nobody but you."

Ed picked Pedro up on his back with Repete following and slowly went to the house. Aunt Lourene saw us and hollered, "Pedro git all that dirt off your shoes." Pedro hollered back, "Aunt Lourene I ain't got on no shoes." We cleaned up and then that day in 1947 came to an end.

Yes, Ed. Pedro did remember. On that day in 1979, Pedro picked up the hoe and shovel, lifted his head, raised his voice and once again sang, "Love Lifted Me."

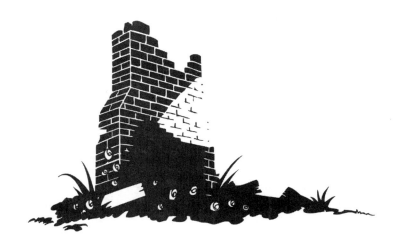

Thangs Worth Fightin' For

I look back on my life and see it entangled with the past — with the loves, the loyalties, the heartaches, and the good times of a large family. Through the years and through the tears, many of them have gone on one by one. Some of 'em gave their lives in World War II so Pedro, Pat, and their young'uns could live in peace. I am still thankful for those I still have.

After the 9/11 terrorist attacks, I upped and decided to ride around the area of the old homeplace. Many of the homes were run down and some were no longer standing. Places where no one lived anymore where so many good times were had. Nothin' there but an old chimney and old roses. The flowers stood and told stories of the old homeplaces.

I continued my journey by some cotton fields where I used to pick cotton until my knuckles bled. The house was still standing but showed its years of wear, and a board was loose on the front steps. The screen door had holes where children had pushed against it in years past. The holes had little wads of cotton poked in them.

On the front porch sat an elderly lady on a swing. Her face was wrinkled with age and was brown like leather from the weather. Her hands were bony and wrinkled like dried apples. She wore a clean apron, which covered the front of her flowered dress. Her eyesight was almost gone but she managed a smile.

I stopped and told her that I was Pedro and that I used to pick cotton for her. I told her I was now a doctor in Tallahassee. A tear of joy fell down her leathery, weather-beaten face and there was an outpouring of love.

As I continued to ride throughout the county I remembered seeing lightnin' bugs in the corn fields at nightfall, smelling the growing corn on hot summer nights, waking up at the crack of dawn with the crowing of a rooster, hearing the church bells ring on a Sunday morning, and seeing the smile of a small child on Christmas Day.

Moultrie was small enough you were never far from thangs and you could come to care for them. If you did, you would find that it was hard to live in peace without them. Some people have died in wars fighting for them. Because they did, we who are their legacy have been given the opportunity of growing up in towns we love in the greatest nation in the history of the world.

In small towns, we learned to love the rustling of corn, the sight of a white cotton patch, the shadows of a quiet street by the courthouse square in a way which made them part of us wherever we went. This, and all the people I have known and cared for, is what I have in mind when I say I love this country and we should defend this country.

An old man once said to me, "I've been everywhere there is to go and I've done everything there is to do. There's nothin' better than what's right here."

I used to wonder what he meant by that. Now I'm willing to fight for that.

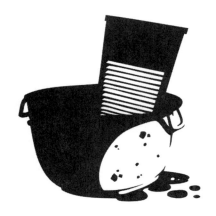

A TRIBUTE TO
MISS CARRIE

M iss Carrie was black. She had been good to me when I was a kid. She was a credit to her race. The human race. She had a better character and was more forgiving than most of us. She loved the South and she loved Pedro.

I waited in the churchyard until everybody had gone into the church. I didn't want anybody to see me if I cried, so I sat down on the last pew. I'd git emotional at funerals, especially if it was somebody who had been good to me when I was a kid.

She always wore a bandana around her head and most of the time her apron pocket kept her snuff and some goodies for us young'uns. She cared for my youngest sister when Mama got sick. One time she held my hand when I fell down and cried.

She didn't have a husband or any close kin and was nearly eighty-five years old. Living alone was hard for a black lady growing up in the South. All her life she lived in the country. Picking cotton in the hot summer months, tending her garden, milking her cow, feeding her chickens, churning and cooking. She loved to cook and she loved to eat and she loved her collard greens. Her country ham with red-eye gravy was the best.

The upper part of her arms were four times bigger than the lower part of her arms and they shook when she laughed, and she laughed at Pedro's stories.

Her house was always clean as a whistle. Dirty rags never spent a night in Miss Carrie's house. One time, a neighbor said, "Miss Carrie, yore house shore is clean and I don't know how you do that." The neighbor was right. She didn't know how Miss Carrie did that.

She always found time to wash clothes and boil them in a black wash pot on the outside. She sang hymns as she did her chores around the house. She also found time for us young'uns.

She kept some dogs, which were mixed breeds like most dogs in the South, and when she called they came running with their noses up in the air. They loved Miss Carrie.

The preacher came in and my mind came back to the little white country church. My eyes noticed the casket. It was silver with white handles. She was dressed in a beautiful blue dress, which was her favorite color. Her hair was as gray as an aluminum cooking pot and she seemed to be smiling. The preacher then said, "Now, let us pray."

The silver-headed preacher said something about finding comfort and strength in the hope that there is life beyond what we know. He said something else about a home on the other side of the river and a home where the streets are paved with gold.

Some friends then carried her through the church doors, and we made our way through the churchyard to a tent that stood over an open grave. As I looked at the hole in the ground, I was reminded that life is only temporary. We know this early in life, but somehow we keep it to one side of our brains.

We then sang, "When the role is called up yonder, I'll be there," and the preacher said a final prayer. I felt a tear when the dirt made a loud thud on her casket.

All the people and all the cars left, and I walked slowly to mine. The sun was setting behind the pine trees. I heard a noise and noticed three dogs running out of the corn fields with their noses up in the air. They headed straight to the fresh dirt and I shivered as the sun went down.

Miss Carrie, a new grave, Pedro, and three lonely dogs. The chapter closed on another wonderful life in South Georgia. She held my hand for a little while but she'll hold my heart forever.

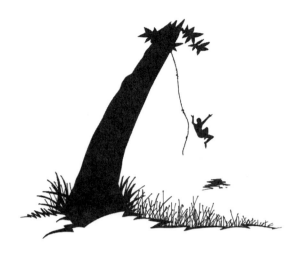

THE OLE SWIMMING HOLE

There are times my heart aches to go back and take my place by the ole swimming hole. In my mind, I know I'm only a stone's throw away, and in my mind I can still sit down by the creek and just think and even go for a swim.

The two best places for skinny dipping and baptism in the north part of Colquitt County (still considered southern by most) were at O'Neal's wash hole and the river bend at Swift Canteen. One could get pleasure for the body and food for the soul. Those days were filled with fun, love, hugs, and smiles.

We always knew it was the right time of year to visit the swimming hole when the whippoorwills started calling and the honeysuckles started blooming. We had already gotten our dose of castor oil, taken off our long-handled underwear, and started goin' barefooted. The corn fields had gotten as hot as Tallahassee asphalt and it was time to cool our heels in the ole swimming hole.

On the way to the swimming hole we'd pass by the blackberry bushes and scuppernong grape vines. This always reminded me of Mama's jelly.

She made jelly so good she could've gotten paid for it, that is if she really had wanted to. She'd rather make jelly than eat, and Mama loved to eat. Her jelly sandwiches were better'n her cold collard sandwiches, or just about.

We'd rush down to the creek remembering that Mama told us never to go into the water after a meal. Mama was right. We never found one. We'd grab a scuppernong vine and swing out over the water and drop off with a blood-curdling yell better than Tarzan, especially if girls were watching. Some of the boys would sometimes sneak off to the creek without permission. They didn't ask 'cause they wanted to go swimmin'. There, they stripped and dipped.

Out by the ole swimming hole out in the open hot sun, Pedro picked up a few freckles. If he could've just pulled them all together, he would have had the best tan in all Colquitt County. Sometimes it would get so hot and the swimming hole so dry the catfish got freckles, or at least speckles, and we called them speckled cats. One time it got so dry that someone said the catfish had gotten ticks. Pedro hadn't fallen off no turnip truck yesterday, so he didn't believe that.

On Sundays the swimming hole became different, with ladies in their long dresses and men in their coats and ties standing on the banks singing "Shall We Gather at the River?" Others were led down to the water for submersion of the body and cleansing of the soul. When they came up out of the water, people said "hallelujah" and the preacher said important things about everlasting life, or at least it seemed important. They then stood there dripping like wet hens and the people did more singing about being washed in the blood of the lamb. People hugged and people cried and again important things were said.

The preacher said that we had left undone many of the things we should have done and that we had done many of the things we shouldn't have done. A prayer was then said and the folks went home. Once again, this place reverted back to the ole swimming hole and a boy's playground.

The ole swimming hole still holds a special place in my heart. It brings back recollections of Simpler Times, when little things translated into big moments and big memories. Those moments and memories, as most things, have continued to grow bigger with the passage of time.

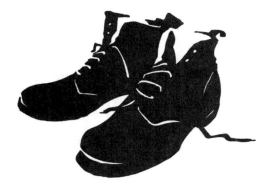

LESSONS OF CHILDHOOD

I often close my eyes and remember the lessons of childhood. They remain as clear as if I heard them yesterday. There is no fence around the memory of time.

Mama tried to help Pedro in his childhood to prepare and get ready for the hardships, disappointments, challenges, and realities of adult life. Mama wanted Pedro to keep learnin' and benefiting from his experiences throughout childhood. She said that we're never too old to learn something stupid. She said that it was OK to dream dreams, but a person needed to be willing to pay the price to see them come true. She told Pedro that it was smarter to plow around a stump than through it and that weak things would become strong if we stuck together.

Mama knew that she wouldn't be with us kids forever and she took every opportunity she had to share her feelings and express her opinions. Mama spent a lot of time around the supper table telling Pedro about life, growin' up, and manners. She told Pedro not to eat with his fingers and never to talk with his fork. Mama spent a lot of time talkin' about politeness. She asked Pedro, "Which piece of chicken do you want?" Pedro replied that he wanted the biggest piece. Mama then pointed out that Pedro should be polite and take the smallest piece. Pedro then asked, "Mama, should I lie or be polite?" Mama said that we'd talk about this later, but we never did.

Some memories stand out more than others. As a kid, Pedro's most favorite dogs were Pete and Repete. They were one-tenth chow and nine-tenths something else. They weren't purebred, but they were from a nice neighborhood and they loved Pedro. The dogs and Pedro chased squirrels together. It hurt Pedro deeply when Pete got killed by a rattlesnake and Pedro cried. It was one of those wipe-your-tears-and-blow-your-nose type days. Emmett said, "Pedro, I wouldn't cry like that if I were you." Pedro replied, "Emmett, you can cry any way you like, but this is the way I cry."

On that day, Pedro did not play. It was hard to have fun with tears in your eyes. It was tough to play hide-and-go-seek or do anything that was fun when you can't see through your tears. Mama said that sometimes little boys are given dogs for a little while so they could learn about life, about death, about growin' up, and about becoming strong. She said that Pedro was her little man and that it was OK for her little man to cry. She said that some things we can never prepare for. That's the way that she had it figgered.

One of Pedro's biggest lessons came at age eleven. Pedro remembered it well 'cause that was the year he got glasses — the ones that kept the big boys from hittin' him and the girls from kissin' him. However, the big boys were laughing at Pedro's right foot 'cause the sole of his shoe was loose and flapping. When Pedro got home from school, he asked Mama why he couldn't get gifts like new shoes like the other kids. Mama wudn't able to speak. She put her cheek next to Pedro's cheek and Pedro felt a tear. It belonged to Mama. She was only able to give Pedro the greatest gift of all — her love.

With all those hardships of childhood and all those lessons of childhood and all those preparations of childhood, Pedro knew he would grow up and be strong. It only partially came true. Pedro grew up. Pedro got grown and Mama's gone. Still Pedro cried. Mama was right. Some things we can never prepare for.

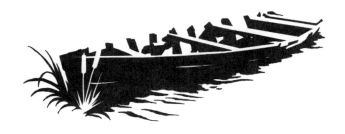

PEDRO AND MILLARD
GONE FISHIN'

D ad called. He wanted to go fishin'. We hadn't been in years but I was too busy and told him we would have to make it another time. We hung up and I couldn't put it out of my mind and this started me to thinkin'. What if there's not another time? Besides, Dad's health was not what it used to be so I called him back and said, "Let's go." He was beside himself. He was so excited. I thought he was going to cry and he sounded like a kid again. Pedro had got grown, got busy, and hardly had time to go fishin' or spend any time with Millard. That's why this trip meant so much to Dad.

When Pedro was a little boy, Millard spent weeks gettin' ready for a special fishing trip to Florida. He would check and recheck the cane poles. He would cut a stob, drive it into the ground, and start grunting for worms. By rubbin' the brick bats across the stob, this would create a vibration causing the grunt worms to crawl out of the ground to be picked up for fish bait. All this we did together. We would then grab some soda crackers, potted meat, sardines, Moon Pies and RC Colas and head to Florida all the way down to Tallahassee to Lake Jackson, always trying to catch the moon just right. In the mid-1940s we would rent a boat at Miller's Landing on the other side of the church for fifty cents and spend the night on the banks or in the car. For a young boy this was livin' in high cotton.

On November 11, 1993, I picked Dad up and headed once again back to Tallahassee. There we were — just like old times, Millard and Pedro, a father and son, except now the father was seventy-five and the son fifty-three and except now the son had to bait his own hook. This time I must have felt what he used to have felt when he took Pedro fishin'.

We finally got settled in and had been fishin' for an hour or so when this young boy came up and asked us how many fish we caught. We replied, "Nothin' yet." He then said, "Y'all doin' as good as the people who fished here all day yesterday." We said, "Yeh, and we're also havin' fun." We then remembered that one time me, Millard, and Dillard fished all day long and didn't catch one single thing. On the way home we stopped by Knight's Fish Market one block off the courthouse square in Moultrie. Dillard asked them to throw him five or six big ones over there where he was. They repeated, "Throw 'em?" He said, "Yeh, so I can catch 'em. I may be a poor fisherman but I ain't no liar."

This day had passed rather quickly between Millard and Pedro. Not too much had been said but the feeling was there. The fishin' had been good but we didn't catch much fish. One small nibble caused us to sit there with each other all day. Hope is such a wonderful thing. There's something special about fishing that brings a son and his dad together, locks out the rest of the world, and makes special memories. Dad had done this for Pedro. Now I got to do it for Dad. This opportunity had almost slipped by and had almost become a memory that never was. Over the years Pedro had growed up and had almost forgot there's more to fishin' than fishin'.

THE BASEBALL GLOVE

Pedro wanted a baseball glove. He wanted it real bad. He wanted it more than anything else in the whole world. He promised Mama and Daddy that if they would give him the glove, he would never ask for anything else and his behavior would improve. Dad looked at Pedro with hurt in his eyes and said that times were tough and the glove would have to wait. However, Pedro knew that he could never be happy again without that glove.

Dad subsequently got sick and became thinner than Pedro and Mary Alice put together. He couldn't shake the memory and problems of the big war where he had received frozen feet and a bleeding ulcer during the Battle of the Bulge. He didn't talk about it much, but you knew it was on his mind. They decided to take him to the VA Hospital and he told Pedro to stay home and look after thangs. He told Pedro to say his prayers ever' night so Pedro could go to heaven. Pedro replied, "I don't want to go to heaven. I want to go with you."

When Dad arrived at the hospital, they decided to give him blood and take out most of his stomach. When Pedro heard about this, he stood there like a little man trying to act brave on the outside, but scared on the inside. Pedro learned that you could hurt real bad on the inside and not shed a tear on the outside. Home was supposed to be where Daddy was, but he was not there. Pedro had trouble sleeping, even when it was time to get up. He thought that he might not see Dad again and he had things to tell him. Pedro was hoping that if it's not your time to die, even the doctors can't kill you.

Word came back that Dad had endured and was coming home. Grandma fell to her knees giving thanks. Mama started shelling peas, skinning taters, shucking rous'nears, and dressing chickens for his arrival. She placed a bright colored piece of oil cloth on the table with some Black-eyed Susans in a Mason jar in the center of the table next to a kerosene lamp with a new wick.

A whole passel of folks dropped by to greet Dad and to howdy and shake and give thanks. As we all sat around the table bonding in laughter and love, Pedro felt secure again and realized that the best things are felt in the heart. The kerosene lamp in the middle of the table casted a glow on our faces as we shared food and closeness. Sitting at that table all gathered together symbolized unity again and, somewhere along the way, Pedro forgot about the baseball glove.

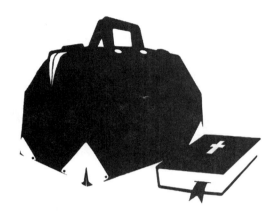

Pedro, Ticks, and Survival

Me and Pat upped and decided one summer to gather up our young'uns and grand young'uns and head up to North Carolina to the mountains to do some hikin' and playin' in the creek. On the eighth day I developed a flu-like syndrome, except it wudn't, and decided to head back to Tallahassee. I was seeing little spots in my eyes and someone asked me if I had seen a doctor. I replied, "No, jest those little spots."

Later, upon arrival in Dr. Judelle's office, he didn't like the way I looked and called the EMTs and sent me to the intensive care unit. My dad never liked the way I looked either but he never sent me to the hospital.

Somebody said I was in septic shock and I could hear Dr. Judelle repeating, "Charles, Charles, speak to me, speak to me," and I cudn't. However, I was thinkin' my reputation is going to pot.

They told me my blood pressure was 70/40 and my oxygen saturation was around 82. They started IV rocephin and gentamicin as well as IV dopamine. They said there were some EKG changes and that I needed a heart catheterization. I was wondering if I really needed that because they might find something.

I could see the concern and caring in Dr. Judelle's eyes and he called in Dr. Gredler who also showed the same concern and caring. I started wondering if I should have any say so or if a doctor's doctor doctored according to the doctored doctor's doctrine or if the doctor doing the doctoring doctored the other doctor according to his own doctoring doctrine. Since I was sort of out of it and I didn't have a choice, they doctored according to their own doctoring.

Dr. Gredler skillfully did the heart cath and told me it was still ticking and that my coronaries were clean. This pleased me greatly but I still didn't want to die in such good health.

Dr. Judelle called in Dr. Nicholson who suspected a tick ailment called ehrlichiosis, which shares some features between Rocky Mountain spotted fever and Lyme disease and has been fatal in some cases. IV tetracycline was started and within twenty-four hours there was a cleansing of the body and my vital signs stabilized as well as my rosacea. Five days in the ICU at TMH was quite an experience and the physicians, allied health professionals, and hospital personnel were wonderful.

After discharge, Dr. Bailey told me that ehrlichiosis wuz a status disease or an elite disease and that only rednecks got it. At least Pedro wuz in good company. At first Dr. Bailey seemed to be an authority on ehrlichiosis but later I come to realize he was actually an authority on rednecks. He said that bathing on Saturday nights would help and Mama told me the same thing when I was a kid and she didn't even go to medical school.

I appreciated all the phone calls and folks who visited me and expressed concern. Dr. Ray was one who tried to visit me in the ICU and had difficulty getting in. I told them that he was my brother and they let him in. He actually is my brother at work and if I could have had a brother he would certainly have made a good one.

When one is laying around in the ICU one has time to think and can learn some valuable lessons. Like, salt is what you don't notice until someone doesn't put it in your grits. Like, you may not recognize the real value of a true friend, your family, and your wife until you are about to leave this ole world. Like, you may not recognize fun in your life and work until it's about to vanish from you. And like, when you are not responding to medical therapy, you turn to a higher power.

There was a whole lot I could say about survival. There was a whole lot I could say about the love of family and friends. There was much I could say about my doctors and caregivers and there was so much I could say about spirituality, faith, and higher beings. However, Pedro is just so happy to be alive and is so happy to find out that there were others who felt the same way.

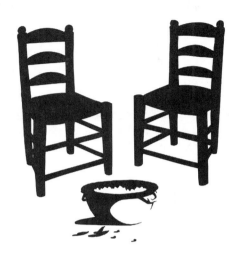

THE FRONT PORCH

While traveling down Highway 319, I noticed some folks sittin' out on the front porch and my mind drifted back to the front porches of Simpler Times, which was a place for gatherin' and makin' memories. It was a place where folks could get out of the hot sun and cool off. One could sit, rock, swing, swat flies, shell peas, and watch it rain. Neighbors and families could gather and talk about those who died, those who didn't, and those who should have. Here, Pedro heard the grown-ups talk about their religion and their government.

On the front porch there always seemed to be enough time for ever'thang and there were more hours in a day than we actually needed. The pace was slow enough that a kid could sit and dream and make plans for the future. The front porch gave a kid a place and time to imagine, ponder, pretend, playlike, and evolve. It was such a good place to ponder and occasionally we pondered so hard we hardly had time to think. Other times we would jest sit and do nothin' and become as worthless as a dead possum tail.

Pedro would sometimes sit on the porch and pretend that Grandma would live forever, that Daddy wudn't have to work so hard, and that Pedro would grow up to be a doctor. He would pretend that he caught the biggest fish in all of Colquitt County and his picture would come out in the *Moultrie Observer*. However, one time Pedro and Millard did go fishin' and came home with some little ones. Millard told Grandma that he almost caught the biggest one in the whole pond, but he got away. Grandma smiled and turned to Pedro and asked, "Is Millard telling us the truth?" Pedro gave a grin as wide as a watermelon rind and said, "Yes, ma'am, and I almost caught one bigger than that."

Kinfolks would come and gather on the front porch and one time when Aunt Ethel and Uncle Arthur were coming, Mama told Pedro to come on inside and wash his face. She said that Aunt Ethel would never kiss him with a dirty face. Pedro, who always appeared to be busier than a barefooted boy in an ant bed, replied, "That's what I thought, too."

It was not uncommon for kinfolks and neighbors to sit on the porch discussing and reflecting on their religion. Most of 'em were Baptists and one time one of 'em said that it was about time the Baptists got to pick the Pope. The Catholics had had him long enough. They asked Hazel if she had ever been Catheterized. She responded emphatically and said, "Of course not. I'm Baptist and I'm goin' to stay Baptist."

Among the men folks, the talk would invariably shift to the weather, how dry things were, their crops, and whether it would ever rain. Once, they told Dad that his corn was awful yella' and little. He quickly told them that he had planted the little yella' kind.

The most heated arguments centered around politics. Dillard told 'em that he had heard that you could lead a man to Congress, but you couldn't make 'em think. Grandma overheard the talkin' and said that Mr. Rogers said that we ought to be grateful that we didn't get all the government that we paid for.

The front porch brought families together and helped children develop their values, their thoughts, and develop their dreams. We all sat around entertaining each other and learning from each other. This was our gatherin' and thinkin' spot. I can still remember Mama and Daddy and the kids sittin' on the front porch watching the sun go down, hearing Mama give thanks and counting her blessings that we were all together, in good health, and had plenty to eat.

The front porch is almost gone now. We lost the front porch to air conditioning and television, but we really lost much more.

The front porch made very special memories. Even with the passage of time, I can still close my eyes and see Mama walk out on the front porch at night and hear her once again ask, "Are all the children in?"

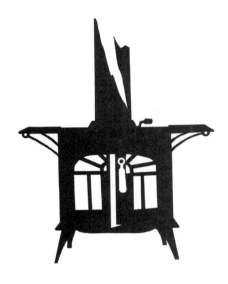

THE BLESSINGS
OF HARDSHIP

Hardships sometimes are a blessing and we don't know it at the time. The good life sometimes deprives us of special moments and we also don't recognize it at the time.

It helps us to look back to our past so we will know how far we have come and it helps our young'uns and our family to know where we have been. Winston Churchill once said that the farther backward you can look, the farther forward you're likely to see.

When I go walking in my mind down the country road of memories, I often remember the hard times on the farm. It has been said that you'd go to sleep with the chickens, git up with the rooster, work like a horse, eat like a pig, and git treated like a dog. Someone once asked a farm boy when he got drafted how the Army was. He replied, "It's real good. The food's good, the work's easy, and best of all, they let you sleep late."

Hard times didn't keep farm folks from being happy. The happiest folks don't seem to be hunting something to make them happy. The government can't make you happy or better off if you don't want to be. The government once sent somebody down to South Georgia to teach a farmer to farm better. He told 'em, "I don't need your help. I ain't farming now nearly as good as I know how."

Even though times were hard on the farm, we had some conveniences, such as fresh milk. We kept our milk fresh by keeping it in the cow. If our milk had been any fresher, it would have been grass.

We didn't have central heat, but we would huddle around the fireplace to keep warm. This brought us closer together and allowed us to share our lives, our dreams, and our thoughts. Mama would knit and tell stories. Dad would whittle and Pedro would do his homework. Keeping warm kept us in the same room and we all listened to Mama. Mama once said, "Pedro, when you git grown and if sickness overtakes you and you ain't got a penny to your name, there's a Mama and Daddy waitin' for you by the fire at home." She said that Pedro was special and that each one of us was unique just like everybody else in this world. She said that we all have an equal chance to be unequal. Often Daddy would just keep quiet 'cause he felt flies couldn't enter a closed mouth. He knew that even though the rooster would sometimes crow, it was actually the hen that delivered the goods.

One night when the fire had died down and it had gotten late, Mama asked Pedro to say his goodnight prayers. Pedro bowed his head and said, "Dear Lord, bless Mama and Daddy and make them happy, if they're not too old for that sort of thing."

When folks got better off and got their central heat, their phones, and their personal TVs, they all headed off to their private rooms and their private worlds. The family was never so close again as when they huddled together around the fire to keep warm.

It seems that hardships brought us closer together and that conveniences and the good life have spread us apart.

Someday I may just throw another log on the fire, turn off the central heat, turn off the TV, unplug the phone, and invite my dad, my sisters, and my family back home again to git warm one more time.

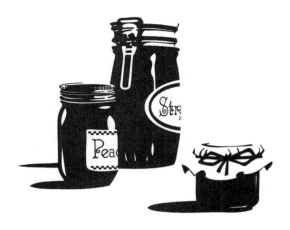

THE WHIPPOORWILL

Over the years, many memories have faded but the memories of Grandma, the old homeplace, and the call of the whippoorwill still remain. These things may be of the past, but they live on in my memory. Grandma seems to be the link to our family's past and our link with each other.

Grandma had gotten old and slow but she said you're never too old to learn something stupid. She pointed out that the worst thing that could happen to ya was the worst thing that could happen. Grandma was humble and poor but she taught us that being poor was not a handicap. Entertainment at Grandma's house was cheap 'cause ever'body entertained themselves. Old-fashion fun didn't cost a dime.

Grandpa died leaving Grandma with their seven kids, her pride, a strong back, and a strong mind. Mostly what she ate, she raised. She planted, hoed, gathered, and canned her crops. She lined the kitchen walls with her preserves and canned goods. She scrubbed clothes on a washboard, cut dress patterns out of paper, and pressed clothes with irons heated on a wood stove. When it was cold enough so the meat wouldn't spoil, she butchered hogs. She did her share of lifting, scalding, scraping, and grinding, and nothing was throw'd away. A supply of lard from hog fat was stored. She saved some of the hog grease to make soap, which was mixed with lye and turpentine. The turpentine kept the worms out.

During the Depression, Grandma didn't have time to get depressed. She was busy raisin' her kids. Grandma and her boys — Millard, Dillard, and Willard — struggled and worked together and laughed and cried together. They had to make a dollar any way they could when they could. They gave each other support and comfort. Love and tenderness helped most folks through the toughest of times. Difficult times seemed to glue the country folks together.

As her family grew, and those of her brothers and sisters, so did the family reunions. One of the most favorite pastimes was sitting on the porch figuring out how we were all kin.

There was always time for sitting on the front porch listening to the whippoorwill. One time, Dillard had been sitting on the porch counting cars. He had already counted three and it wudn't even dark yet. Grandma reminded him that he wudn't make much money doing that. Dillard studied on it and replied that he wudn't spending much either. At the end of the day, someone pulled up in the yard and asked, "How do you get to Claude Bennett's store from here?" Grandma replied, "Sometimes I walk and sometimes Dillard takes me in the truck."

On the day of rest, folks dressed up in their Sunday best, which was usually the same outfit as the previous Sunday. The community and a higher power was a pillar of strength during hard times. During dark days, neighbors, friends, and family were there for comfort and their presence gave a special kind of care when it was most needed. That's the way Grandma had it figured, and I figured she was right.

People come and people go and the old homeplace is no longer standing. Even though Grandma's gone, her memories still pull my heart toward home and give me comfort, and the whippoorwill still calls.

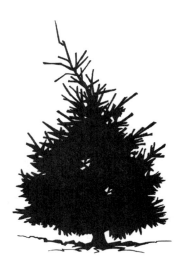

Mama's Prayer

When Christmas comes around in the air, my mind turns to the Christmases of Pedro in Simpler Times. In South Georgia in the 1940s, times were lean as Christmas approached. Men tried to make do for their families and would accept any kind of work. In those years, our folks told us not to expect a whole lot 'cause Santa was hard up too. We had been warned that Santa had to spend his money on food for the poor. So often us young'uns went to bed with heavy hearts, hoping for a miracle and wonderin' if Santa Claus would come. When you grow up expectin' less, any kind of gift was received with joy.

We would start early decoratin' for Christmas and place strands of colored lights on the front porch of our shotgun house. It was three rooms deep and one room wide. It looked desperate but sometimes a few bright lights seemed to make a difference.

We would walk through the woods to find the right tree, and the right tree always seemed crooked. The tree was propped up in the front room, which was the kids' sleepin' room. The tree was then sprinkled with salt and flour to make it white and sparklin'. Paper chains and colored buttons were hung on the tree. The paper chains were held together with paste made with a little flour and water. This was our tradition, and even back then I was big on tradition.

During the past half-century, I've been very fortunate in my life to have received many wonderful gifts. However, the gifts I remember the most are the ones that had a lot of thoughtfulness behind them and the ones given to Pedro in Simpler Times.

One of Pedro's most favorite gifts came during the Christmas of 1948. On Christmas Eve of that year Pedro went to bed with his shoes on. Mama said, "Pedro, you can't sleep in bed with your shoes on." Pedro replied, "It's OK, Mama. They're not my good ones."

After Mama and Pedro said their good night prayers and after Pedro's spankin', Mama tucked Pedro in.

Pedro kept wonderin' if Santa Claus was comin' and had trouble goin' to sleep even though he was plum tuckered out. He knew Mama and Daddy had not been shoppin', and they kept tellin' Pedro that this had been a hard year for Santa Claus. Pedro was 'bout worried as a Christian Scientist with appendicitis. Pedro wanted some toys.

'Bout midnight, Pedro got up to go to the outhouse. It was so cold he could see his own breath, and it was colder than a tombstone in January. He noticed smoke comin' out of the chimney and when he got back he stood in the doorway quieter than a sinner in church. As Pedro stood there, he saw Daddy makin' a sling shot out of a hickory stick by the light of the fireplace and noticed Mama kneelin' down on one knee by Daddy's side. Pedro could barely hear Mama's voice as she spoke with her head bowed. Mama was sayin', "Help Pedro to understand that times are tough and we love him dearly. And help him to understand the meaning of Christmas and that he is our special gift and maybe through some miracle we can also be his." Pedro backed out of the door with a lump in his throat feelin' the greatest love that he had ever known. Pedro went back to bed thinkin' that on Christmas morning he would receive the greatest gift of all: Mama's love.

On Christmas morning, Pedro woke up with a joy in his heart and remembered "Mama's prayer," best expressed in an old hymn:

Tho' years have gone, I can't forget
Those words of love – I hear them yet.
I see her by the old armchair,
My Mama dear, in humble prayer.
When-e'er I think of her so dear,
I feel her gentle spirit so near.
A voice comes floating in the air,
Reminding me of Mama's prayer.

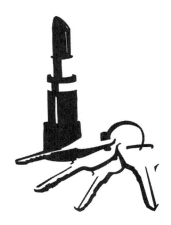

DRIVING, DATING, AND HURTING

Dating in Simpler Times was not exactly simple, but it was exciting, filled with humor and clumsiness, and sometimes associated with hurt. Romance was often seen through rose-colored glasses and when hurt did occur, youth had the ability to quickly rebound and heal.

Mama told Pedro's sisters and cousins that the way to a man's heart was through his stomach. Once, Hazel, who was in her teens, was visiting the homeplace at suppertime. We usually had beans and taters and some nights we had taters and beans, but on this night we were having liver. One good thing about liver was that you could always get enough of it. A good-looking young man from the Norman Park community dropped by and Mama told Hazel that it was OK to ask him to stay for supper. Hazel then said to him, "The weather's bad and you'd better stay and have some liver with us." He replied, "Thank you. I'm much obliged, but the weather ain't that bad."

One could not do any serious courtin' without a driver's license and a car. In 1956, Pedro and the 1949 Ford had a few problems. Pedro had starter problems and sometimes overheated. The car had door problems and the door on the passenger side had to be tied shut with haywire and the front seat rolled forward when you hit the brakes. Pedro and that car circled the courthouse square in Moultrie, Georgia, so many times looking for girls that the price of gas went up.

One could not properly date without a driver's license and the state patrolman only came to Moultrie every two weeks to give the test. Upon turning sixteen, Pedro couldn't wait. Mama reluctantly gave in and took Pedro to Thomasville to take the driver's test. Upon receiving his driver's license, Pedro took a quick look and said, "Mama, if I look like my driver's license, I'm too sick to drive back home."

Pedro will never forget his first real date all by himself. He was real nervous, but Mama told Pedro just to be himself if his date could put up with it. When Pedro arrived at the door to pick her up she was actually prettier than a speckled puppy.

Pedro and his date headed to the Sunset Drive-In. Upon arrival, he put the speaker on the window and got settled in. The people in the next car over were giggling and making loud noises. Pedro felt that anybody having that kind of fun had to be sinning. Pedro then remembered that the preacher once asked, "What must you do before you can expect forgiveness of sins?" Someone in the third pew shouted back, "You must sin." Pedro felt like he needed to be real careful 'cause people in Moultrie were able to hear the news before it never happened.

After the movie, Pedro headed to a dead-end road near Ballard's dairy farm off Thomasville highway where there was a lot of dirt between the houses. When he got there, there were already a lot of other cars. Some folks called this Lovers Lane. Pedro put his arms around his date and she said, "Don't kiss me. I got scruples." Pedro stopped. He did not want to catch the scruples. He knew a lot of Baptists with scruples and it stayed with them most of their lives. After a while the police arrived and people started leaving like ants in a burning log.

When Pedro got home, Dad asked "Where have you been most of the night?" Pedro told him that he had been riding around with the guys. Dad replied, "Well, one of the guys left his lipstick in the car."

During the night, Pedro had it figured out that he had fallen in love. Next day he went by to tell her that he was not worthy of her love. He didn't get the chance. She told him first. Pedro's heart was aching. His lips felt numb and there was something in his throat. He didn't know if he could make it to the driveway with all that hurt, but he tried. As he was leaving, Pedro decided to look back for the last time, and for the first time he noticed that she had big ears.

Note: Colquitt Regional Medical Center now sits on the old Lovers Lane.

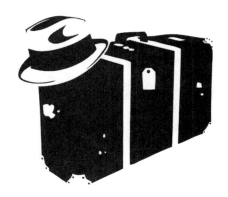

FRIENDS AND THE JOURNEY OF LIFE

S ome of the best antiques are old friends and I visited with some of my old friends and fraternity brothers one weekend at St. Simons Island. These were the people I had lived with, studied with, and played with during my undergraduate studies at Mercer. Most I had not seen in thirty-five years. I pulled out my old fraternity blazer and it had shrunk. I then pulled out my jersey and it had also shrunk. This had been a good weekend. Nothing is wasted that makes happy memories.

I saw friends and faces that had been so dear to me, but the years had gone by and some could no longer be with us. As we gathered on this day and as I looked around the room into those faces, the reality set in that time really does pass. After a while, I did not see judges, lawyers, other doctors, teachers, and business people. I saw friends. I saw family. I saw a part of me.

We had all been on the same train ride thirty-five years ago heading to our individual goals, but the true joy was the trip and the true joy was what was happening along the way. We all had initially started the train ride with the same fears of tomorrow. If I had it to do over, I would have stopped counting the miles and watched some sunsets, studied harder on my second organic chemistry test, gone barefooted more, had more laughter, and spent more time with my friends and appreciated them more. You just can't seem to make it up in one weekend, but I tried.

Upon arrival for the weekend I saw Pope Hamrick and Bert Carmichael. Bert had become a chaplin and Pope was a judge in Daytona Beach, Florida. Bert had a bet with Pope that I wouldn't be there. Dick Porter, an attorney from Cairo, Georgia, kept the money. At the banquet that evening I was requested to present the money to the winner. I took the opportunity to talk and talk and told them that I didn't want to insult any of my fraternity brothers, but I heard that many of them had become attorneys. I also knew most of 'em when they were first admitted to the Bar, long before they attended law school. I assured them that I supported attorneys and most of my medical colleagues supported attorneys. I recommended that they send their own children to medical school, so they could also support attorneys. The two lone doctors in the crowd clapped. I then gave Judge Hamrick and Chaplin Carmichael their money back with special instructions that judges and preachers shouldn't be bettin'.

We returned to our tables and Pope reminded me that John Parks, now an attorney in Americus, Georgia, had been his roommate, but John was not exactly tidy in those days. One day, Pope called a conference between himself and John, instructing John that they were going to divide up the room for cleaning purposes. Pope then asked John, "Which half of the room do you want to clean?" John replied, "I'll take the top half."

Another story was then told about Jerry Vanderhoef, another judge who was from Alabama, and Phil Addy, a farmer from Preston, Georgia. In their college days Phil decided to take Vanderhoef home with him for some dove hunting. Upon arrival Vanderhoef exclaimed, "I don't have a hunting license!" Phil explained, "We don't need any. It ain't hunting season." Later Vanderhoef shot a real nice big white one — a pigeon.

As the stories were flowing, David Sims, one of my best friends, told us about Dean Knight's wife. Mrs. Knight was driving on the sidewalk across campus to pick up Dean Knight outside the Knight Building. It was raining. As Mrs. Knight approached, David and Pope stuck up their thumbs hitchhiking even though they were only going another fifty feet. To their surprise, she stopped and picked them up. As they proceeded down the sidewalk in Mrs. Knight's car, they approached Granger Rich, a blind fraternity brother, coming down the same sidewalk. They warned Mrs. Knight that he was blind and that she should stop. They let the windows down and David asked Granger if he wanted a ride. Granger stuck his head in the window and said some ugly words about driving on the sidewalk that only upperclassmen would understand. David quickly let the window back up and said, "Mrs. Knight, we don't know who that foul-mouthed person is. He must be a Sigma Nu." Mrs. Knight smiled and said, "Dean Knight is a Sigma Nu."

It was fun telling each other old stories. However the real fun was seeing each other and being next to each other one more time. We continued to exchange stories and memories. We talked about old times and good times. We talked about what we had done and should have done, but didn't. As we were talking, time went by and the weekend, just like the past thirty-five years, creeped upon us and came to an end. We hugged and smiled and went our separate ways, hoping for all of us another tomorrow.

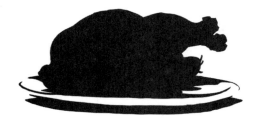

Memories
of Thanksgiving

With Christmas on its heels Thanksgiving so often doesn't get its due. However, on Thanksgiving Day, Pedro comes closer to the memory of his roots than at any other time. Thanksgiving was a time for us kinfolk to reflect back on our upbringin', our values, and our raisin'. Such memories had a way of retaining their flavor as we fondly recalled the warmth and love that always surrounded us at Thanksgiving in Simpler Times.

Kinfolks (the young, the old, the strong, the weak) came together for eatin' and closeness and for reflectin' and rememberin'. All were cherished by the family. It was a time for giving thanks and sharing feelings.

Folks who had moved away came back to visit family and friends and to think about those who have passed on and whose influence still remained. We dropped by the cemetery to honor Grandpa and those who were no longer with us and decorate their graves. At that moment, life seemed so precious. Life seemed to start and end with the family. It made us feel so proud to have lived in Simpler Times and in that place.

In the ole days, Millard, Dillard, Willard, and cousins by the dozens came together to share food and stories that could be passed down through the generations. It was our memories of who we were, where we came from, how we got there, who's buried where, and who married who or should have but didn't. Fond memories were made with food and togetherness.

Folks brought black-eyed peas, turkey and dressin', mess o' greens with ham hock, collards, corn on the cob with real melted butter in between the kernels, and more food than we could imagine. One time after a hog kill, Dillard brought some chitlins. He said that you just don't eat anybody's chitlins. You needed to know who done the washin'. Anyhow, food tasted better back then before we found out about cholesterol and when fatback, eggs, and sunshine were good for ya. The food was always good but Mama said that all food was good if you waited long enough. When we had tripe, I guess we just didn't wait long enough.

The central gatherin' spot was the porch or the kitchen dependin' on the weather. That was before television and it was hard to want something you never knew. Television would have messed up our discussions but at least young people nowadays know more about deodorant and detergents than any other generation.

There'd be mixin' and minglin' and laughin' and talkin'. Pedro heard about guns, crops, fishin', women, government, and hard times. When grown-ups were talkin' we kept quiet and listened very slowly. At these gatherin's we heard about hard work and learned how to get dirty and come up smilin'. Grandma wanted us to be happy and she felt like the happiest folks weren't always hunting something to make them happy. However, the teenagers felt like they needed a car to pursue happiness.

Eventually discussion led to religion. Even if folks had stole hogs, got drunk, told lies, and cheated, they were always thankful they still had their religion. There were many folks who felt people needed the Bible for the soul and liquor for the spirit but Grandma was against liquor. Her idea of happy hour was a nap. Grandma wanted Pedro to be nice and to be good. She once asked Pedro, "Where do little boys and girls go when they sin?" Pedro replied, "Out behind the barn."

Thanksgiving always brought back warm images of people we loved and of times we loved. Our folks had worked so hard that they didn't have time to get rich. Thanksgiving allowed us to escape for a day from a world that was on the way to becoming so complex and so manipulated, but on this day we had remembrance for the past and hope for the future.

At the end of the day ever'body would be plum tuckered out and the dark would start moving in to any place it could find between the lights. On this day, thanks would be given and troubles forgotten.

It had been a good day but Grandma said that any day would be a good day especially if you were around to make it so.

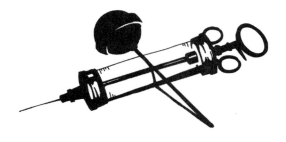

Dreamin' On
The Front Porch

As a kid, I would sit on the front porch thinkin' and dreamin'. That's where we did that. Sometimes just me and my two dogs, Pete and Repete. I could depend on them to keep my secrets. Sometimes I would play what it would be like. What would it be like if ever I could become a doctor, what would it be like the first day of practice, what would it be like the first day in the operating room, what would it be like the first time I could fly in a real airplane, and on and on. Just what would it be like?

My first day in the operating room was not what I had envisioned in my youth in Simpler Times. No heroics. I was assigned with two other junior medical students to observe Dr. Gramling, anesthesiologist at Medical College of Georgia. As a junior student, it was obvious that I, along with my two classmates, didn't know what was going on. Dr. Gramling was giving a local anesthetic to the mental foramen of the mandible and apparently blocking the nerve to the mental foramen. He looked at our name tags and mine was the name he could pronounce. He said, "Dr. Williams." Then I froze, I had never been called Doctor. It didn't seem right. It still don't seem right. He then said again, "Dr. Williams." And asked, "How do you do a mental block?" I thought and thought for about ten seconds and said, "Dr. Gramling, I know but I can't think of it." He stopped, took off his gloves and went around to every room repeating what some junior medical student had told him. Later that day I was getting more and more confident and was assigned to observe Dr. John Williams do surgery. He was a first year surgical resident and apparently his job was to cuss and my job was to run and get blood. We both did our jobs well.

The first actual day of practice was in the Pediatric Department at Homestead AFB, a long way from Moultrie and a long time from Simpler Times. On this first day an Air Force Sergeant brought his five-year-old child in for his vaccination. There was a bottle of lollipops on my desk for rewards. I reached for a lollipop with one hand and had the needle and syringe in the other. The Sergeant's kid looked my way and said, "I don't want any of your damn lollipops. Just give me that shot and let me get the hell out of here." I did just that and I ate the lollipop. By the end of the day all the lollipops were gone.

The first day of practice had finally come to an end, but there was the sound of some soft footsteps. Upon turning around, there stood a cute little five-year-old girl dressed in a pink princess outfit with a crown. She sweetly said, "Trick or treat." I had forgotten it was Halloween and the lollipops were gone. There were a couple of oranges on the desk left over from lunch. She opened her sack and I dropped in an orange. She looked into the sack and looked back up at me about to cry. I thought that was not enough. I reached for the second orange and dropped it into the sack. She again looked into the sack and pitifully back up at me. I asked, "Weren't the oranges enough?" She replied, "You crushed my damn cookies." This had not been exactly the dream I had on the front porch back in Simpler Times and since that day I've heard of others with a similar experience (E.G. Pinyoun).

After two years of Pediatrics, Pediatric Radiology became appealing and I flew to Houston, Texas, to start their program. On the way out there, I got one of the seats right by the window so I could look out during my first airplane flight. It seemed that a lot of my dreams from Simpler Times were being fulfilled. After several hours of flying and looking out of the window, I turned to the gentleman sitting next to me and told him that we were finally over Texas. He said, "How come?" I said, "'Cause the pine trees are getting taller." He looked over me and out the window and said, "No they're not, we're landing."

Upon arrival I went over to Texas Children's Hospital to hear Dr. Singleton, Pediatric Radiologist, give a conference to approximately a hundred physicians. He had written an article called, "Dwarfs and Other Little People." He was presenting a case of an achrondroplastic dwarf and said that this mother had six other children just like the one presented. He then asked if anyone in the audience knew this family. I raised my hand and asked if her name was Snow White. He stopped and asked me who I was and where I was from. I told him Moultrie and he said, "That explains it." He subsequently received a Gold Medal Award from Pediatric Radiology and became my mentor and friend.

After entering the world of private practice of Pediatric Radiology, one evening I got a call from Dr. Jordan, the orthopedist, about doing a hip aspiration using fluoroscopy on a four-year-old male child to rule out infection of the hip. He said the Pediatrician would be giving orders to the nurse for proper sedation. About forty-five minutes later, I entered the room to perform the procedure. The little boy was lying on the table with his eyes closed and absolutely no movement and the mama and grandma were standing by his side. I proceeded to explain the procedure to his mama. I told her about sticking a needle into the hip joint to get fluid using x-ray to help guide the needle to the right spot and that the fluid would be sent to the lab for tests. The mama appeared a little faintified and queasy so I asked, "Does anyone wish to leave the room?" The little boy opened his eyes, looked up at me, raised his hand and said, "I do." I then left the room for more medication.

Many of these actual happenings weren't exactly like the dreams formed during Simpler Times, but those dreams gave some of us young people hope and direction. The dreams on the front porch allowed us to leave the front porch and prepare for a more complex future time. During these present complex and hectic times, I find that now my dreams take me back to the front porch of Simpler Times for peace of mind.

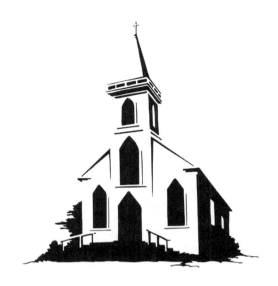

PEARLIE'S PASSIN'

A unt Pearlie passed away day before yesterday. She went to join Willie. It was unexpected. It usually is. We weren't prepared but we usually aren't. It was hard on ever'body.

Lots of folks poured in, some from way off and most of 'em Pedro hadn't seen in years. They all brought food and nobody was hungry or was gonna be. They all said nice thangs about Pearlie and they all said she had suffered enough. They all said she'd be missed. Then we all headed for church.

There it was: Hopewell, the purty white church on a hill. One could see through the corn fields the grammar school Pedro attended. As Pedro stood there on the church grounds overlookin' the corn fields and gnats, he remembered thangs. As he looked over to the school, he remembered Aunt Pearlie smilin', clappin', and cheerin' as he got on the school bus for the first time in 1946.

Pearlie was the great encourager. She was the head cheerleader. Pedro remembered when he graduated from Moultrie High, Pearlie was there. She clapped and hollered. Pedro remembered when he graduated from college, Pearlie was there. She clapped and cheered. Again Pedro remembered when he finished medical school, Pearlie was there. She cried.

Pearlie weren't never on television and Pearlie weren't never in *People* magazine and she hardly ever left Moultrie. Yet Pearlie was a very important person and the world never knew it. Too bad. She made the people who knew her feel important – even Pedro. She made him feel like he could make good grades, do his numbers, and maybe even become a doctor if he studied hard enough. She told Pedro to go off and git some learnin' but not to act uppity when he got through. She also told Pedro to treat old folks with respect, to look out for snakes when he went blackberry pickin', not to mess around with gopher holes, look out for sandspurs, don't chew with his mouth open, don't smack at the table, warsh behind his neck, keep on a clean change of underwear, be good to your neighbor and they'll be good to you, and keep on the sunny side of life. She said to take time to stop and smell the flowers but to remember that you can't smell a rose if you got a fungus up your nose.

One time, Pearlie told Pedro that we were here on this earth to help others and Pedro responded, "What are the others here for?" This stumped Pearlie and she didn't know. She said, "I reckon we'll find out when we get to Heaven." I reckon she now knows.

Pedro continued to think about Pearlie while standin' outside the church waitin' to go inside. He remembered one evenin' at suppertime over at Pearlie's when he was tryin' to cut his meat and he was about seven. Pearlie looked over at Pedro and asked, "Are you sure you can cut your meat?" Pedro replied, "Oh yes. We have it this tough at home all the time."

Pearlie and Willie had been Dr. Paulk's tenant farmers for several years. They had a fish pond out back just beyond the pecan orchard and the bean patch. Pedro lived just a short piece down the dirt road and one day he sneaked off and went fishin' without askin' Mama, Pearlie, or Willie. They all discovered Pedro wudn't around and started a big search and found him at the fish pond. Pearlie then asked, "Pedro, if you wanted to go fishin', why didn't you come and ask me and your Mama first?" Pedro responded, "'Cause I wanted to go fishin'." Me and Pearlie had a lot of memories and I knew a sermon couldn't do justice for Pearlie and it didn't but it was a good sermon.

We then sang four hymns, the same hymns Pedro and Pearlie used to sing shellin' peas on the front porch and in the same order. That's the way she would have wanted it. Pedro felt somethin' in his throat when they sang "In the Sweet By and By" and "Precious Memories."

Pearlie will be missed but she will not have lived in vain. The Pedros of the world have become better off from having known and having been influenced by the Pearlies of the world. If your Aunt Pearlie is still livin', go see her. Tell her she is appreciated. I wished I could.

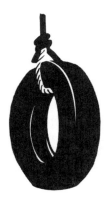

SWINGS AND THINGS

I was layin' on my back on the porch in Bradfordville with my toes up in the air drinkin' sweetened iced tea in my wife's finest crystal and callin' the dogs when my mind drifted back to Simpler Times. Some of the pleasures of that time seem lost forever to videos, television sets, and air conditioning.

One of the pleasures back then was swingin' and doin' nuthin'. It seems that just being has not been given its just due. The quiet hours I spent swingin' remain etched in my memory. It gave a young boy time to dream, reflect, hope, and prepare.

I learned about my family and their history on the porch swing shellin' butter beans and shuckin' corn with Mama, Aunt Pearlie, Millard, Dillard, and Willard. We'd sit together cuttin' the corn off the cob while tellin' stories and laughin'. It gave us the chance to be together as we felt a closeness and it gave Mama the opportunity to give Pedro direction, guidance, confidence, and hope for the future. We must have swung a million miles.

As we sat there on that swing, Mama said that it's what's on the inside that counts and makes us what we are. You can cover it with sugar, put it in the stove and cook it, and call it something else, but a cow pile is still manure. She pointed out that some folks think they're worth a lot of money just because they have it.

As we would swing, Mama said that ever' young kid needs to git ready for life and eventually ever' wash tub has to set on its own bottom. She would give Pedro hugs and tell him to hold his head up, to toughen up, and never to give up. She told Pedro to reach for the stars and that edukashun would help. She didn't want Pedro to be illiterate like Hazel's son down the road. Someone once told Hazel that her son was illiterate. Hazel replied, "That's a dad-burned lie. My son ain't illiterate. I was married almost three months before he was born."

We weren't exactly second-class citizens. We had two swings. The second one was an old tire that hung by a rope from a tree limb. Pedro spent many hours sittin' in that tire with his feet pumpin' him to the sky. As Mama pushed and Aunt Pearlie clapped, Pedro imagined being able to touch the stars with his toes. Mama reached out with her love as she told Pedro to keep reachin' for those stars. That helped a no-good country boy to feel good about himself.

When Pedro started to school wearin' those homemade flour sack shirts, Mama's words helped Pedro to overcome the teasin' and still feel like a somebody. Pedro needed that. The memory of Mama's words and Mama's hugs helped Pedro through some mighty tough times.

Now-a-days whenever I pass down an ole country road and see a tire hangin' from a tree, I want to stop, find a kid, give 'im a hug and tell 'im to reach for the stars. That kid might need that.

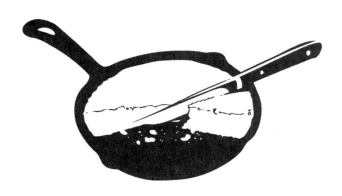

DISAPPEARANCE
OF SOUTHERNERS

I was trying to figure how to sign off my radiology reports on the computer and Drs. Yaakob and Killius (both from New York) walked by and I said, "How y'all doin'?" I realized they looked puzzled. I then realized they needed help in gettin' educakated on how to act in public and how to properly talk. I also realized Southerners in Radiology Associates of Tallahassee are a disappearing breed and this seemed to be happening all over the South.

I then went to the books and according to a study of ten years of research at the University of North Carolina, the number of people living in the South who identified themselves as Southerners dropped by 7.4 percent during this timeframe. As with other parts of the country, urbanization and migration are having an impact in the South and there are a bunch of folks from way up above Atlanta coming down this way. Most of 'em are pretty good people, like Dr. Moore, and some of 'em have taught me a whole lot.

To some of these folks, Southern accents sound uneducakated and perhaps make some people thank the speaker is a bit slow. However, many Southerners can turn that accent on and off at will and use it to their advantage, pouring it on when they want to feign ignorance, luring the unsuspecting into a trap.

Whether it's the backwards sound of my daddy from the cotton fields of South Georgia, the sweetness of a Savannah drawl, the slow cadence of Dr. Patty from Southern Mississippi, or the unique sound from the hills of Robbinsville, North Carolina, my ears perk up and I want to know where they are from and how they got there. Part of being Southern is the accent, the phrases, and the sayin's. "Lawdy, Lawdy, Lawdy ... ," I can still hear my mama blurting out dozens of times a day. I also remember Mama telling Daddy, "No use trying to fix that ole wash pot. It's plum wore out."

In the South we certainly had our sayin's that is to yore ears what chicken fryin' on Sunday is to yore nose. I remember back to the Simpler Times when words of wisdom were funny, when family wuz ever'thang and money wuz nothin', when folks weren't too uppity to laugh at each other and themselves. We'd never call anyone crazy. Instead we'd say, "Her cornbread ain't quite done in the middle."

What concerns me about all this and gives me sadness is the homogenization of American culture. As the number of people who consider themselves Southerners declines, so too, I suspect, do those who consider themselves New Yorkers, Northerners, etc. Our distinct differences, instead of being celebrated, are melting away as we all move about and mix and watch the same television, see the same movies, shop at the same stores, and wear the same clothes. Pretty soon we'll all be talking the same way and our uniqueness will disappear.

Now when I take a notion to go back home in South Georgia and visit with Aunt Pearlie and Uncle Willie, Millard, Dillard, and Willard, I listen closely. I appreciate those sounds, sayin's and accents even more 'cause I know all too well that some day they may be gone away forever and the Pedros of the world will all sound and act the same. Lawdy, Lawdy, Lawdy, I hope not.

This has been the beauty of America and we've been the melting pot for many cultures and races and all this has been part of this grand country called America. I hope we can still maintain our uniqueness. In the meantime, I'll continue to talk the only way I know how. Hope y'all have a great day now, you heah?

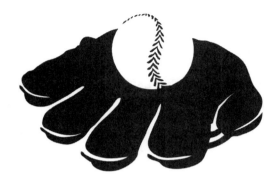

BEST THANGS IN LIFE

As time goes by, my memories are being more and more shaped by my heart and I carry them with me in the life that remains.

During my life, I've witnessed many changes, and as a kid we were poor but the government at that time wasn't coming around telling us we were poor. I've been part of what we call progress. I remember our icebox being replaced by a refrigerator at age seven, our outhouse being replaced by indoor plumbing at age eleven, getting a party line telephone at age fourteen, and getting a black and white TV with snow as a late teenager, but the TV didn't have a chance to mold and control my life. I remember picking cotton from daylight to dark for three dollars a day and being replaced by a cotton-picking machine.

With each generation there has been more advancement and gadgetry. We now have CDs, computers, beepers, faxes, web sites, truck phones, and the list goes on. We have answering machines to screen calls and call waiting so we won't miss a call from somebody we didn't want to talk to in the first place. Folks are even out there creating animals in the laboratory and folks are going to the moon. By the way, Grandma thought going to the moon was fake and wrestling was real.

It seems that everybody's life is getting more complicated. The other day I received a fax from the Florida Radiological Society, an e-mail from the American College of Radiology and a call on my home phone from the hospital when my beeper went off all at the same time. I got in my truck to hide and my truck phone rang. It must have been more peaceful in the days of the Pony Express.

Sometimes I think I work for a computer. I no longer can do a barium enema examination if the computer is down. I can't perform a BE unless it is on the computer. I can't dictate a report unless I have a form from the computer. The report can't go out until I sign off the computer.

Things keep advancing and things keep changing and progress continues to be made. Twenty years ago audiocassettes were on the cutting edge and now they are outdated. In another decade all the things that complicate my life now will be outdated. I wonder if we had been doing surgery first for poor eye sight and then glasses were invented whether folks would be rushing out to get glasses so they wouldn't have to have surgery.

In spite of all of this, I am grateful that all thangs have not changed. Still nothing beats the smell of a log burning in the fireplace, the taste of homemade ice cream on the Fourth of July, the change of leaves in the fall, roasting marshmallows and wieners on an open fire, walking barefooted down a dirt road, chasing fireflies at night with yore grandchildren, walking down the beach and holding hands with yore wife, and cane pole fishing with yore dad at the creek. Note: If you are too busy to go fishing, you are just too busy.

But even if we continue to make progress and all my gadgetry breaks down, I can still say goodnight prayers with my grandson and watch him throw a baseball.

As much as I can tell and as much as thangs have changed, so much has stayed the same. The best thangs in life are still the best thangs in life.

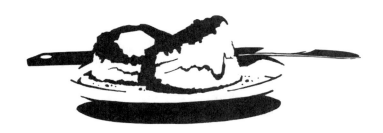

BARE FEET AND BISCUITS

I no longer live in the country, but thanks to my childhood the country still lives in me.

After the passing of winter, a country boy's feet start itching to be set free from his shoes, and I was thankful that going without shoes was stylish in the spring and summer for country folks in Simpler Times.

In my day we didn't need Nikes or Reeboks to win races. The winners of races were barefooted and this gave them an edge. They would jest dig their toes into the dirt at the starting line.

It was unusual for kids to git new shoes in the warm weather. In the 1940s we'd git a new pair of shoes right before school started and right after the crops had been gathered. They had to last all winter. Our most favorite pair always seemed to be the most cheapest. We could not wear them until it started turning cold.

Mama said that our shoes needed to last a long time and going bare-footed helped our shoe budget. She also said that being poor didn't make you handicapped.

Many times before spring arrived, the soles would start flopping and Mama would stretch the shoe budget by refastening floppy sole shoes with glue or screen tacks. When the shoes got tight from growing feet, a slit would be made to give relief. She said that I had to tell her where to make the slit because you have to wear the shoe to know where it pinches.

One time holes developed in Pedro's shoes in the wintertime and they were beyond repair. Pedro asked Mama, "Why can't I have some new shoes?" Mama didn't say a word. She grabbed Pedro and hugged Pedro. Pedro felt a tear on his cheek. It belonged to Mama.

Uncle Dillard, who was Millard's and Willard's brother, decided to take Pedro in to be fitted for a brand new pair. The salesman asked, "Where will these shoes be worn?" Pedro replied, "On my feet. One on the right and one on the left." Dillard then smiled and I thanked him. Over the years I have thanked him over and over in my heart.

Sometimes when Sunday mornings came around and it was time to hear the preacher talk and find out what Hell was really like, we'd pull out our shoes. There was no polish. We'd rub our shoes with a cold leftover biscuit. I think it was the lard in the biscuit that gave them the shine.

In the spring, after the call of the whipporwill, after the sunning of the mattresses, and after our dose of castor oil, we shedded our shoes and our feet started toughening up. We'd walk barefooted through the plowed fields and it felt better than any foot massager. I was so glad to set aside my outgrown patched shoes for toe freedom in the dirt. My feet loved the dirt but my feet wuz somewhat like my hair. When I washed 'em, I cudn't do a thang with 'em.

Even now, when the whipporwill calls and the weather starts warming up, I git the hankerin' to shed my shoes and spread my toes. I also git an itchin' to go to a set-down restaurant to sop biscuit and gravy and then, dadgumit, the sign on the door says "No Bare Feet."

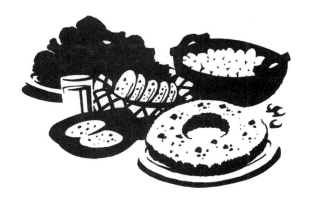

MEMORIES
OF CHRISTMAS

Christmas is just around the corner and memories will be made. The joys of this Christmas will be tomorrow's memories and precious memories will linger with us.

Most of us have a rich treasury of Christmas memories from our own childhood and so often we continue customs from our own heritage. I have wonderful memories of Christmas in Moultrie and very few have anything to do with money or material things. I remember the feelings of this season and things that money can't buy.

Christmas for Pedro began on the day school let out. That was the same day of the Christmas play where Pedro got to play the donkey, except for the one time they used a real donkey. That was also the same day the Off-Key Children's Gospel Group sang "The First Noel." The program was heavy on scripture, prayers, and Christmas carols. That was before the Supreme Court ruling.

The main attraction in Moultrie was the strings of Christmas lights on the courthouse square leading up to the sky to the top of the courthouse. A star towered above the lights reminding us of another star more than two-thousand years ago.

There were memories of going with Daddy into the woods to select and cut a perfect tree. The perfect tree always seemed crooked. We'd drag it home and decorate it with paper chains and other homemade ornaments. Aunt Pearlie always said that it was the prettiest tree she had ever seen.

The magic of Christmas always carries me back to the unheated bedroom of my childhood. I remember pressing my face against the cold glass of the bedroom window while covered with two or three quilts hoping to catch a glimpse of Old St. Nicholas' sleigh and reindeer dashing among the stars. Sometimes I still glance up to the heavens on Christmas Eve looking for St. Nick. I've never seen him in flight, but I've seen the magic he leaves behind.

Mama said that Christmas was not about money. She said that Christmas was about love and caring. That's what Mama said. It seems to me that we do a lot of unusual things at Christmas to reflect that love. It also seems that we don't understand how to express it so we go to Wal-Marts and Stein Marts trying to find the perfect gift, which turns out to be somewhat less than perfect.

Some of the most precious memories are those spent with family. My family and I have been so blessed at Christmas but I feel saddened that so many children will not have the opportunity to experience the kind of Christmases that many of us have seen and felt. There are many children who have never known the joy of wishing for something special and then finding it under the tree. There are also children who have never known the joy of giving to someone else.

One of my most favorite Christmas memories came about when I was about eight years old. There was a family who lived a short ways down our dirt road. The father had been ill and out of work. We wrapped and loaded up some of our old toys for distribution later. Mama had baked some cakes and cookies. She also dressed and fried some chicken and made an ice-box fruitcake. Daddy had picked up some pecans from the yard and we headed over to their place in our old Ford coupe.

I'll never forget the excitement of those kids. It's been over fifty years now and I don't even remember their names. However, I'll never forget their faces and the tears in their mama's eyes. I wish all people could know the special feeling that Pedro felt during that Christmas at that time.

Still, there are families even in Tallahassee who are doing without this year at Christmas. Still there is plenty of time.

Merry Christmas to all.

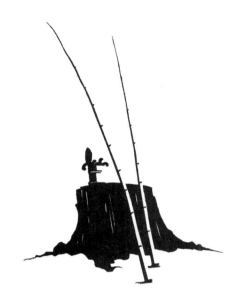

Goin' Fishin' and Catchin' Love

When I was a kid, being a kid was hard, but bein' a good kid was even harder. Times spent fishin' with Dad helped Pedro git through the hard times and to grow up. The simple pleasures that us young'uns got from fishin' down at the creek with Dad were abundant and kept us out of trouble. When you didn't have a whole lot, it was easier to appreciate some of the finer thangs of life like fishin' and spendin' time with the family. Even now, when I'm fishin' with a cane pole I come closer to the memory of my Dad than at any other moment.

Dad realized that life was short and realized what was precious in life. Dad said that fishin' helped him to relax even though some folks seemed to be the happiest when they were uptight and miserable. For Dad, fishin' and spendin' time with us young'uns seemed to give a meaning to his life.

On one of our good gettin' up mornings, we picked up some grunt worms and gathered our cane poles, homemade tackle, and a small fish net, which was a lot of little holes tied together. We loaded all this on our truck — and our truck was a real truck. It didn't have the non-essentials like a muffler and windshield wipers. It was a truck that didn't require washin' and that nobody would steal.

On the way to the fishin' hole, we stopped by Dillard's and the smell of his pigs almost keeled us over. Pedro asked, "Don't the smell of all those pigs bother you?" Dillard, who seemed as happy as a pig in a mud puddle replied, "Sometimes, but it just depends on the price of pork."

Millard then asked Dillard if he wanted to join us fishin'. Dillard smiled and said that today he just felt like spendin' the day with Elizabeth Taylor again. Millard said, "Again?" Dillard replied, "Yeah, I felt like it once before."

We went on to the creek and Dad told Pedro to be real quiet. He told Pedro how deep to fish and where to wet his line. Dad was so smart and Pedro felt so loved and safe.

A barefooted boy who was ugly as an empty glass of buttermilk came by and started talkin' to us. His sinuses were so bad it was hard for him to talk through his nose like the rest of us, or either he was from up North. He said that we would do better if we fished with flies. Pedro then told him we *were* fishin' with flies. We also had been sittin' with flies and eatin' with flies and sometimes even with gnats.

As we sat on the banks of the river, Dad talked about his life. He said, "Pedro, life is full of uncertainties, I think." He said that when life gets hard we need to keep our head up, toughen up, and hunker down. He told Pedro never to sass Mama, never to point in public, to be good to old folks, and other commandments that he had learned from his mama, who was Baptist and knew ever'thang.

So often we didn't catch fish, but the fishin' was always good. Many times our lines got caught in the trees and Dad would say, "Y'all fishin' for squirrels? Y'all will never catch any fish in those trees." And we didn't. More importantly, we did catch plenty of love. Thanks to Dad.

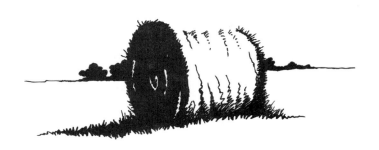

A Whole Lot
About Nothin'

I was running late getting to work. I had run out of Total cereal and had to eat twelve bowls of that other stuff. I was trying to be my colon's best friend. This put me behind and put me to thinking. Having time to do nothin' has not been given its full due.

It seems that many of us are so busy and responding to what is happening at the moment that we don't have enough time to do nothin'. We find ourselves working hard and making good time but we don't know where we're headed and we miss out on the simple pleasures of living.

I noticed this past summer that even many kids didn't have the chance to do nothin'. They were being taken to swimming lessons, ball practice, music lessons, and the list goes on. Their entire days were filled. They were so busy trying to respond to their parents' wishes and trying to please their parents that they didn't have enough time to simply enjoy being a kid.

Summers aren't spent doing nothin' anymore. Summertime has become almost as hectic as the school year. Summer activities seemed to begin before the school year has ended and perhaps some of these activities do have some value.

I wonder if while we strive to provide our children with every available opportunity, we are causing them to miss out on something else — the simple pleasure of living. The pleasure of living without obligations or schedules, the pleasure of enjoying moments as they come and just being a kid 'cause there isn't anything more exciting to do.

All of us miss some things from our own generation. In my time, the freedom of a country boy was endless and we used it. We used our imagination to occupy ourselves and entertainment didn't cost a dime. Any day could be a good day but it was left up to us to make it so.

Wouldn't it be wonderful having a summer of doing nothin'? Days doing whatever struck our fancy. Days hanging out with your best friend — in my case, my wife.

It's so easy to close my eyes and open up a wandering mind and see events of my summer childhood: taking off long handles, going barefoot to toughen up my feet and save the wear and tear on my good shoes, watching Mama air the mattresses with sunshine, chasing mosquito hawks, noticing tall fragrant pines, smelling bacon and eggs and a pine scent in the crisp morning air, hearing blue jays squawk their good mornings, and walking down a country road in the summer and smelling newly mowed hay. The scents, sounds, and sights of summer — what memories and images they evoke.

On lazy afternoons sitting with Grandma, there wasn't much to disturb the tranquility except the angry scolding of blue jays. Their call will always remain a link to sitting in a rocker on the front porch with Grandma as she shared her memories and her past. She passed along family traditions, shared wisdom and moral values, and showered us with love to last a lifetime.

Back in Simpler Times there was plenty of time to appreciate your surroundings, plenty of time to talk to your family and friends, plenty of time for your parents to listen and hear your concerns, and time to daydream and ponder and decide what kind of person you wanted to be when you grew up. There was time to decide what kind of road you wanted to travel down in your life.

These opportunities to do nothin' allowed a kid to use his or her imagination and dream and even figure out who he or she is and where he or she is going.

Even as adults, doing nothin', allows us to appreciate the simple pleasures in our own life and to figure out what we want in the remainder of our years and if we need to change direction. It allows us to get refreshed, refueled and ready to do something.

We're all so busy — both adults and children. Still, we all sometimes need time to do nothin'. There's one problem as I see it: It's hard knowing when you're through.

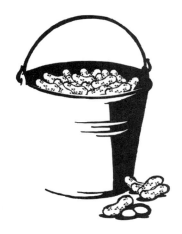

Pickin' on Rednecks

Nowadays, it seems the only group that people can pick on and not be considered politically incorrect are those of us raised in the South and referred to as rednecks.

People such as Jeff Foxworthy have made fortunes talking about rednecks. He says that you're a redneck if the Salvation Army ever declined your mattress. He also says that a redneck considers a pick-up truck with lawn furniture in the back to be a limo.

However, all rednecks ain't bad. Many of them have risen to great heights. At least a couple are listed in Ripley's Believe It Or Not — one for being an only child and the other for having liability insurance on his truck. Believe it or not, at least one redneck has become a doctor.

Sometimes I think rednecks have been given a bad rap and folks need to be educakated.

The term got its start when folks like mine made their living in the fields in the hot summer months trying to grow food for their families and others and their necks became red.

When these country folks, farmers, and sharecroppers went into town on Saturday to git feed, seed, and flour and to see what was happening, city folks noticed that their necks were red. Some of the city folks thought that these country folks were ignorant and uncouth.

These folks drove pick-up trucks that didn't need washing and trucks that nobody would steal. They listened to the Grand Ole Opry on Saturday night and they knew all the words to the old gospel hymns on Sunday. They freely used "y'all" and "ain't" in their sentences. When they wore their overalls, they weren't trying to make a fashion statement.

My dad was one of these folks. He had one of the biggest hearts and he was one of the most kindest and most caring people I have ever known.

In his earlier years, his neck got red walking behind a mule trying to make a living for his family. He was at his best when his hands were in the soil. He didn't know how to read but he did know how to give a dollar's worth of work for a dollar's worth of pay. He also knew how to say "thank you" and "yes, ma'am" and he did give us love. On Saturday night he was standing by the radio listening to Hank Williams on the Grand Ole Opry and on Sunday morning he was down on his knees thanking the Lord.

These folks would take time to sit on the porch with you and visit for a spell. They also took food cooked from scratch to a home where there had been a death and would stay long enough to do the dishes. They would pull off the side of the road when they met a funeral even though they didn't know the deceased. They would go to the cemetery and stand over the grave of a loved one long after the family member had died.

These were people you could trust and people you could count on when you were in a bind. Their handshake and word wuz much better than a contract. They would pick you up when you were down, comfort you in time of sorrow, share with you when you were in need, and tell your mama when you done something wrong. They helped this ole boy git his edukashun.

I'm an offspring of these folks who worked the soil and became red of neck, and I'm proud of it. A whole lot of folks seems to be pickin' on rednecks. I think I'm going to go out to the doctors' parking lot, git in my truck, listen to Hank Williams, eat some boiled peanuts, and sulk.

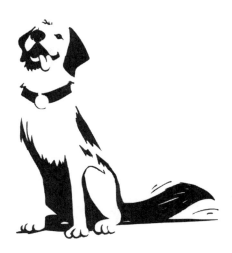

HAPPINESS IS IN THE TAIL

As a kid, I spent a great deal of time fishing down at the creek. Many times, a great big airplane would fly over way up in the sky and I thought I would be happy if I could someday, somehow fly in one of 'em. After I got grown, my wish came true. Now I fly a great deal on behalf of the American College of Radiology as a passenger and now I look down and wish I wuz fishing in the creek.

Sometimes it's hard to explain what made the good ole days good, but over the years I often have thoughts of how happy we were in Simpler Times. Once again, this put me to thinkin' and I started wonderin', what is happiness?

Happiness seems to be different things to different folks. One senior citizen thought happiness was an eighty-seven-year-old man that got married because he had to. Someone else thought happiness was taking your boss to supper and he sat down on the only stool without a top on it.

Other folks think happiness is the absence of problems. I got plenty kinfolks without any problems but most of 'em are buried at Hopewell Baptist Church in Colquitt County. Those that ain't buried seem to have their share of problems.

As I look back I remember how poor we all were, all the problems we all had and, as I recall, my folks seemed happy and somehow nobody got analyzed. It seems that if you're standing under a pine tree and it's falling, you don't analyze it. You just git out of the way.

Hard times and problems seemed to bring country folks together. The happiest people didn't necessarily have the best of ever'thang. They just seemed to make the best of ever'thang.

People shared back then and people cared back then and neighbors helped neighbors and friends helped friends. Many folks seemed the happiest when their heart was beating for others.

Some folks think happiness is getting something. Some seem to think they'd be happy if they had such and such a car, a new dress, a suit, a new boat, and the list goes on. Many of us were led to believe if we'd finish college, get married, get a place in the suburbs on a half-acre lot, mow grass on Saturday morning, and barbecue on Saturday afternoons, we'd achieve happiness.

We set up goals or dreams in our mind that we want to arrive at. Sometimes we achieve these goals but something still seems missing. Other times we never quite reach the goals and they continue to outdistance us. Maybe, just maybe, the true joy is the trip and not the arrival and not the end.

Psychologists have said that an inner feeling of success and of accomplishment will make us a better person, a healthier person, and a happier person, and these intangible results are what make life livable. It is in the little pieces of accomplishments along the way that make for a happy, successful life.

One great source of happiness in Simpler Times was our family and the quality of time we had together. This type of happiness could not be bought. There once was a boy who was born of poverty stricken parents in a poor rural farming community. He married a local girl and had several children. He was a dedicated, hard worker and eventually became wealthy. He sought happiness. He obtained factories, properties, and oil wells. He had a home in Destin, a mountain retreat in the Highlands, and a million-dollar yacht in the Keys. However, he never forgot the poor community where he was raised. Once a year, he went back and visited his wife and children. Still, he wasn't happy.

Someone once told a dog that happiness was in the tail. The dog wanted happiness so badly he started chasing his tail. He went around in circles, never quite catching it. In frustration he said, "Heck with this happiness thang. I'm going to do my own thang!" He started walking off and looked back and his tail was following him. Apparently it was not something to go after but it was one's state of mind.

Abraham Lincoln once said, "Most folks are about as happy as they make up their minds to be." It seems to me that happiness is a journey and not a destination. The really happy man or woman is the one who can enjoy the scenery along the way, even if he or she takes the wrong road. You git to the point too quickly and it ain't much of a point, but the thangs along the way are what really count and may be better than what's at the end. It seems to me that the true joy is the trip and not what's at the end. Happiness apparently is a state of mind as we're making the trip to get to the station.

Forcing oneself to be happy don't seem like much fun. It seems to me that the happiest folks are the ones not always huntin' something to make them happy. If only we'd stop trying so hard to be happy and stop going in circles chasing our tails, we could have a pretty good time.

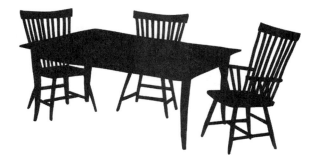

A MAMA'S LOVE

Mother's Day is the day we set aside to honor those who brought us into this world and cared for us.

If your Mama is still alive, go see her. Tell her she is appreciated. I wish I could.

So often we don't appreciate the best moments of our lives and the most important people until it's too late. Life is about change, and today's joys may be tomorrow's memories, but on Mother's Day I'm at least thankful for the memories. We need to pay more attention to the treasures in our lives while we still have them. Mama once said to Pedro, "Enjoy the little things in your life, for one day you may look back and realize they were the big things."

Mama had about as little as anybody I've ever known but I never heard her complain about anything she didn't have. My mama's dresses were handmade and she was glad to have them. She frequently reminded Pedro not to make fun of other people's clothes. She said that whatever a person wore was probably the best they had.

My mama lived through a depression and a world war. She ate buttermilk and cornbread cooked at home in the same old black frying pan. She placed a value on truth and honor. She wanted a brighter future for her son and she delivered.

My mama was a praying woman and I knew this 'cause she walked through the storms of life with her head held up to the heavens. One time she was looking up and I heard her saying, "O, Lord, someway, somehow help my son git the schooling I never got, which he needs to help him on in life."

She listened to my prayers at night and she woke me in the mornings. She listened to my concerns and gave me encouragement. Pedro did not feel very smart until Mama kept telling him he was and then he was.

My mama loved me enough to teach me right from wrong. She loved me enough not to give me ever'thang I wanted. She gave me more hugs than switches but enough of the latter to keep me in line. She made sure I knew the importance of education and that gift has taken me places I never dreamed of. Most of all she gave me love. One time, Mama said, "Pedro, you've outgrown my lap but you'll never outgrow my love."

Some of the best memories I have of Mama were at the supper table. The supper table was the center for teaching values, expressing feelings, sharing, and hearing Mama's sayings. I think we'd all be better off spending more time with our own children at the supper table, even if you want to call it dinner.

Pedro learned a lot from Mama at the supper table. First, I learned I had a place in the family and that I belonged. I also learned to share and had to pay attention to the number of folks at the table so I could take the proper portions. I was grown before I realized the chicken neck wasn't really Mama's favorite piece of chicken.

Mama watched our manners and I cudn't fill my plate until ever'body was seated and the blessing had been said. When you wanted something passed you said "please" and then "thank you."

One time, Mama asked Pedro if he wanted some beans. Pedro replied, "No." Mama said, "No what?" Pedro replied, "No beans." Mama then said that she wanted us to say "no, ma'm," "yes, ma'm," "no, thank you," and "please." She didn't want us young'uns to grow up with people thanking we were Yankees.

Mama's sayings at the supper table still ring in my ears even on this Mother's Day. "Being nice don't cost a thang and is worth a fortune." "'Please' and 'thank you' will take you further than a Cadillac, for a lot less money." One time she said to Pedro, "I know you licked the plate clean but I still have to wash it."

Of all of Mama's sayings, the one I remember the most and that meant the most was "I love you, son." This probably will always be the favorite saying of all Mamas.

On this Mother's Day, I wish with all my heart I could once again go back to the old homeplace, see Mama and say, "I love you too, Mom."

Happy Mother's Day.

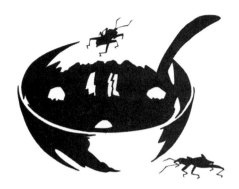

Larry, Stink Bugs, and Turnip Greens

Sometimes large extended families have members who are child-like even when growed up. They are referred to now-a-days as special or gifted. Larry was such a child. He was Aunt Lourene's brother and she and Ed raised him. He didn't have no schoolin' and mostly what he learned was in his own backyard. He done the simplest of all chores, like keepin' the flies off the table food, with great pride and dignity. He was a person of few words but he used them a lot. Sometimes he would pitch a fit and have thirty fits a minute and each one of 'em would last an hour. However, more often than not, Larry was a joy in his child-like way, but occasionally he would git in the way and he'd git sent outside to play hide-and-go-seek. He'd show up an hour or so later saying that he won 'cause we didn't find him.

One day Larry came to spend the day with us. It was the same day the preacher was comin' to eat. This was also the same day a stray bulldog wandered into the yard. Mama hollered out the back door for Larry to quit making faces at that dog. Larry shouted back that the dog started it first.

We just kept a-waitin' for the preacher to git there and Larry started complainin' about his stomach hurtin'. Mama said it was 'cause his stomach was empty and as soon as something was put in it, it would feel much better. Finally the preacher arrived and he said his head was hurtin'. Larry told the preacher that it was 'cause his head was empty and as soon as he put something in it, it would feel a lot better.

We sat down at the table and we were all anxious to start eatin' and Mama called on the preacher to say Grace and bless the food. He must have misunderstood. He blessed us, the weather, the crops, the lost sinner, Larry, and finally the food. His blessing was long-winded and said with the same conviction and vigor of his sermons.

Right smack dab in the middle of the table, Mama dun put a big platter of chicken with the pulley bone belongin' to the preacher — there was a platter surrounded with cornbread, turnip greens, black-eyed peas, and little green onions. The preacher dug into the food and Larry asked, "Are stink bugs good to eat?" The preacher then asked, "Why, Larry?" Larry replied, "'Cause one was in your greens but it's gone now." That didn't seem to bother the preacher none. He kept on eatin'. He was already fat as a hog at killin' time. Pedro kept thinking that if the preacher don't stop soon, we'd be eaten out of house and home. He must have packed it in clear all the way down to his toes. Mama then brought in the blackberry cobbler and the preacher said that this was 'bout as close as we git to Heaven and still have our feet on the ground.

After all that eatin', we headed to the front porch for some sangin' and fellowship. Larry loved his sangin' or just maybe it was 'cause it brought all of us together. Larry loved to see us smile and loved to see us happy and he was part of it. He then wanted us to sang 'bout a cross-eyed bear named Gladly. The preacher reminded us that Larry was referring to the hymn we sang at church last Sunday called, "Glady, the Cross I'd Bare."

I believed Larry enjoyed that day 'bout as much as Mama and Pedro. It felt good knowin' he belonged and he knowed it. During his whole thirty-something years of life, he touched our lives, warmed our souls, and made us laugh. It put me to thinkin' that we all touch people's lives one way or the other, even the Larrys of the world.

That day ended with all of us sangin' Pedro's favorite song, "Precious Memories," and the words still ring loud and clear:

> *As I travel on life's pathway,*
> *Know now what the years may hold.*
> *As I ponder, hope grows fonder,*
> *Precious memories flood my soul.*
> *Precious father, loving mother,*
> *Fly across the lonely years*
> *And old home scenes of my childhood*
> *In fond memory appear.*

In the stillness of the midnight,
Echoes from the past I hear
Old-time singing, gladness bringing,
From that lovely land somewhere.
Precious memories, how they linger ...

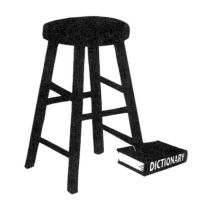

LITERACY AIN'T
EVER'THANG

This, I don't understand. Recently I read this in a newspaper:
"Current market valuations coupled with increasing volatility has expanded option premium and created substantial opportunity in the option market for those investors and speculative risk tolerance and basic understanding of options."

I read it again and again. Still I don't understand.

It seems to me that some folks git educated beyond their intelligence and use big words and hard words to sound uppity and to confuse us. Many of my folks weren't educated but literacy ain't ever'thang and sometimes it complicates thangs. Even though my dad wudn't educated, I did understand him. Once, Dad said, "Since I ain't educated, I'll have to use my head."

What I remember most about growing up in Moultrie was the people and their smiles, their handshakes, their compassion in times of need, and their strength in times of trial. But it was in their simple words that I received samples of their wisdom. There was something remarkable about their understanding of the most complex circumstances. These difficult problems were made simple by just a few simple words, well chosen.

From Daddy I heard: "You're only as good as your word. Trust comes from your hand. You give a man your hand and it's good as done." At least

Dad's word and others like him meant more than all those complicated fancy words you could put on paper or in a contract, and at least you could understand him. These folks with simple words did know about respect, honesty, fairness, and hard work.

Grandma also used simple words and phrases, which have stuck with me over the years. Phrases like: "There's no right way to do a wrong thing," "Play with fire and you git burned," "Whoever lies down with dogs, gits up with fleas," and "When the horse dies, it's time to git off."

I can imagine an over-educated intellect taking a phrase like "Beauty is only skin deep" and saying, "Pulchritude possesses solely cutaneous profundity," or a phrase like "Birds of a feather flock together" and saying, "Members of an avian species of identical plumage congregate," or a phrase like "As the ball bounces" and saying, "Thus is the erractic manner and direction in which the resilient spheroid exhibits its compressive elasticity when propelled against a surface."

"Pek" Gunn, post laureate of Tennessee, once said:

> *Once I used high sounding phrases*
> *But one day at last I found*
> *Truth in story simply stated*
> *Renders it no less profound.*

Once, Daddy said, "Pedro, if you sass your Mama, don't mind yore teacher, and don't do yore homework, I'm goin' to take you out behind the barn and skin you alive."

This, I understand.

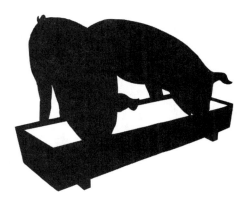

EATIN'

Eatin' sure has changed over the past few years. During the Depression when it wuz hard tryin' to make ends meet, Grandma thought all food wuz healthy, especially when you were as hungry as a starvin' bed bug. Someone once asked Dad what his favorite food wuz and he replied, "Anythang I kin git." As a kid we ate whatever Mama put down and wuz glad to git it. Mama once said, "You put the hay down and the goats will eat it."

During Pedro's footloose and carefree days as a young'un, some folks ate thangs that city folks cudn't find even on menus in big cities. Thangs like possum. Possum wuz best eaten with sweet taters. If you served it with anything else, it would git up and walk off the plate. If you served it rite, even a hunter would come out of the woods to git it.

Possum wuz more tender if cooked twice: once when it's young and again when it gits older. One needed to take extra caution to make sure the possum wuz well done 'cause there wudn't nuthin' worse than being accused of servin' a half-baked possum.

However, the basic meat of country folks back then wuz hogs and when it turned cold it became hog killin' time. After butcherin', they were eaten from snoot to tail and the remaining meat wuz preserved by saltin' and smokin'. We used all the hog including the lard and the chitlins.

Nuthin' was throwed away except the hog's squeal. People were starving in some countries and here we were throwin' away the squeals.

Some folks probably don't know what chitlins are but some of us were born into culture while other folks jest had to be taught. To educate those other folks, chitlins meant hog intestines. An informed country person jest didn't eat anybody's chitlins. They needed to know who dun the washin'.

One time after hog killin' Mama loaded up two #10 washtubs full of chitlins on the back of our pickup truck. On the way home she told Dad to drive careful. She said, "I'd hate to have a wreck and have the doctor try to put all those chitlins back in us."

Another meat item of country folks was fried or stewed rabbit. My family did have their limits and didn't eat rabbit. After eatin' rabbit, some folks kept a rabbit's foot for good luck. However, Pedro cudn't figure out why carrying a rabbit's foot was lucky since four of 'em didn't seem to help the rabbit much.

The best food in South Georgia was Mama's chicken. Nuthin' could beat one of her pullets fried in hog lard with some of her butter beans simmered in a little water with a chunk of pork throwed in. When a yappin' yard dog would come around, a piece of Mama's chicken would shut 'em up ever' time. Her chicken would have made the Colonel weep.

On Sunday morning at sunrise Mama would place the chicken's neck on the choppin' block, and with a quick whack that chicken's head would fall off. That chicken without her head would start runnin' around in the yard faster than anythang you've ever seen. Without that extra weight, that chicken could really move.

We'd try to git by with make-do fixin's. After fryin' chicken or pork you'd leave enough grease in the fryin' pan and add three or four table-spoons of flour and stir to dark golden brown. We'd add a touch of salt, pepper, and water and cook it until it would jest barely run out of the spoon and then sop it up with cathead biscuits ... that is if you felt like it, and we usually did. We'd git filled up and satisfied too.

I don't know what our eatin' back then did to our bodies and it worries me to think about it. I do know what our suppers did for our family, as it brought all of us together.

I look back over the years at how poor we all were and the troubles we had and I believe our gettin' together for closeness and sharing at sup-pertime helped our family to survive those hard years.

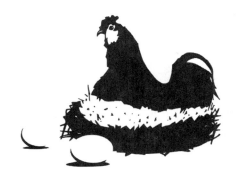

A BAREFOOTED KID
MIGHT BE WATCHING

There were a lot of big days in South Georgia in the 1940s. One of the biggest was the arrival of Dr. James R. Paulk, a young new specialist. He knew everything about eyes, ears, noses, and throats. He settled in and was not only well thought of but was respected. He purchased a farm on the Claude Bennett Road to raise cotton. There were also cows, chickens, and a pecan orchard. He selected my Aunt Pearlie and Uncle Willie to be his tenant farmers. We lived just a short piece down the dirt road.

He would come late in the afternoon to check on thangs and get eggs. At the age of five I quickly figured out his pattern and would come running barefooted with a dirty face behind his new black shiny car. I would remind him that I was doing a good job keeping that egg-suckin' dog out of the hen house. He would pat me on the heard and say, "Pedro, you're a good boy." I believed him. He was the second person who had told me that. Mama was the other one.

I never got to know Dr. Paulk, the man, very well, but the image he projected to me served as a powerful guiding force to an impressionable kid in need of heroes and a sense of direction.

Time passed. Pedro went off to medical school and even graduated. Dr. Paulk had not realized that Pedro and Dr. Williams were the same person. I visited Dr. Paulk after graduation in 1966 and told him I was Pedro, guardian of the hen house. This brought back memories.

He grabbed me and hugged me for two minutes. For a second I thought I saw a tear on his cheek.

Again time passed. In the 1980s Dr. Paulk's wife had a coronary arteriogram at Tallahassee Memorial Hospital by Dr. Allee, and Dr. Jawde did a coronary artery bypass. Dr. Paulk came down to the Department of Radiology to visit. At the time I was doing a femoral arteriogram and was gloved and gowned. They led him into the room. He had aged and his vision was now poor. He placed his face about six inches from mine in order to see Pedro again and he again grabbed me and held me for about two minutes. For a second I thought I felt something on my cheek.

As he was leaving I was thinking I never told him what he meant to me and the influence he had on me. He never knew at the time and neither did I. Will the cycle be completed? Is there a young person out there that I may influence and not know it at the time? Perhaps I should be careful and do better. An impressionable barefooted kid in need of direction might be watching.

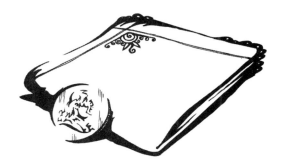

KINFOLKS, HOME FOLKS, AND CHILDHOOD

T here are many people and events that touch our lives over the years. They all play a part. One day we notice we've growed up and something is missing. We then realize it's our childhood and we then find ourselves lookin' back 'bout as often as we are lookin' ahead.

One person who touched Pedro's life was his other grandma, Grandma Murphy. Mama was a Murphy before she married. One time somebody asked Pedro what was his mama's name before she was married. Pedro replied that he didn't have a mama before she was married. Grandma and Grandpa Murphy lived mostly off the land and mostly around Coolidge, Georgia. They were poor and uneducated, but it has been said that literacy ain't ever'thang. They, like most folks around there, were Baptist. There didn't seem to be too much difference between the Baptists and the Methodists. They both sinned, but the Baptists had more trouble enjoying it.

One time when Pedro had gotten home from church, Grandma Murphy was there waiting. She hugged Pedro real tight and asked him, "What did the preacher talk about in his sermon?" Pedro replied, "I don't know. He never did say." Pedro then went on inside, took off his Sundy-go-to-meetin' clothes and put on some hand-me-downs. He rolled up his britches legs, went back outside and started playing in the dirt. Later Mama hollered outside and said Grandma was thinkin' 'bout takin' him home with her for a few days and that he would need to come back inside and get a bath. Pedro hollered back, "Can't we wait and find out for certain first?"

In her older years, Grandma Murphy left Coolidge and moved into the housing project in Moultrie, Georgia. Even to this day Pedro looks back and still misses her. He was there three days before she died. It was late August in 1962. Dog days had set in. Pedro had finished Mercer University and was the only one workin' at the cotton gin with a college degree. Kinfolks were beginning to sit at her place on the font porch. Usually a bad sign. Lights were dim on the inside. Another bad sign. Pedro went inside and she stuck out her weak, frail, wrinkled hands to clutch his. He held them closely and said, "Grandma, I'm going to medical school this fall and it's going to be hard." She pulled out a handkerchief from under her pilla'. Both ends were tied in a knot. She asked Pedro to untie one of the ends and out fell a fifty-cent piece. She said, "It's not much, but I want to help and it's yours." Pedro replied, "Grandma, thank you. Ever' little bit helps and I love you." Even though he had been told this his whole life, it was at that moment that Pedro truly learned that it was not the amount of the gift that counted, but it was the love, thought, and caring behind the gift. Also, at that moment Pedro knew that Grandma Murphy had received a special blessing.

Pedro got a lot of gifts from a lot of folks over the years when he was gettin' his edukashun. Ever' little bit did help and it all added up and a lot of blessings were received.

There were other folks who also gave gifts to Pedro and one that comes to mind is Ms. Godbee. She gave him the most noblest gift of all — herself. She pushed, inspired, encouraged, molded, and guided him and other young people through their childhoods and made Moultrie, Georgia, a better place to live. Some folks called her a second grade school teacher. Mama called her an angel.

Ever' single person, whether they were your grandma or your second grade school teacher, seemed to play a part. Ever' single thang and ever' little bit contributed to make a whole and to make an adult. The days became years, the boy became a man, and the child arrived into adulthood. Pedro can't seem to separate hisself from his kinfolks, his home folks, and his childhood. Sometimes it's a thorn in the side, but most of the time it is a comfort and a source of guidance and strength. Childhood may have been physically left behind but the experiences of childhood persist and can't be separated from the adult. I guess Pedro will always have in him a little touch of Grandma, a little touch of Pearlie and Willie, a little touch of Ms. Godbee and a whole bunch of Millard, Dillard, and Willard.

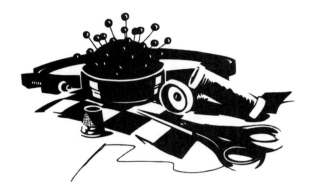

GRANDMA, QUILTS, AND MEMORIES

Pedro had been up at Moultrie visiting Millard when he took it on himself to stop by and set-a-spell with Willard's daughter, Judy. He hadn't seen her in a coon's age. Upon arrival Judy said she had picked up a quilt from over at Uncle Dillard's and Aunt Annie Mae's that Grandma had made for Pedro before she died.

When Pedro saw that quilt that Grandma had made specially for him, it brought a lump in his throat and it put him to thinking. He remembered as a child that Mama would put a quilt on the floor for us kids for afternoon naps. Mama would also put a quilt down for a pallet in the front room when kinfolks and friends came to spend the night. Nobody was turned away as long as Mama had a quilt and a floor. That's what quilts and floors were for.

When Pedro saw that quilt and all those tiny pieces of cloth that had been sewed into a pattern, he knew how hard and how long and how much love she had put into it. She had spent hundreds of hours of work putting together a thang of beauty. Grandma had saved all scraps from makin' dresses and shirts and she had saved all flour sacks and guano sacks. Each piece could even have its own special memory. One piece of scrap could have been from a special Sundy-go-to-meetin' dress or another patch could have been left over from a family reunion outfit. Pedro knew that this quilt would be passed along to each generation and he suspected Grandma knew that too, and that each generation would have remembrance.

When Pedro thought of Grandma, he thought of the love she showed and gave to her family, to her friends, and to Pedro. He thought of her wit and her humor. It was these qualities that brought her family closer together and helped them to overcome tragedy and hard times. He remembered one time on a windy day in March in Colquitt County, someone had asked Grandma if the wind blowed this way all the time. Grandma studied on it and replied, "No. Sometimes it blows the other way."

Pedro continued thinkin' and remembered Grandma's wit and wisdom and she said that we should not cut down the tree that gives us shade and that we should not be all vine and no taters. Most likely what she meant was don't be all talk and no action.

Through Grandma, Pedro learned not to go back on his raisin'. He learned of love and loss, and how fleeting were the moments of our lives. He learned that the most precious thangs were the most simplest thangs and it was the simplest thangs that formed permanent pictures in our memories. Robert Browning once said, "If you get simple beauty and naught else, you get about the best thing God invents." That's what Grandma gave and that was what the quilt reminded me of, and it was mine to keep.

We cannot turn back the pages of time and time won't stand still, but Pedro has his quilt, his memories of Simpler Times, and his memories of Grandma. And "memories are our treasures here on earth." Through telling these stories, it is hoped that Pedro leaves a glimpse of Simpler Times for others to remember and to enjoy and maybe trigger a special feeling, a special moment, and a special time in one's own Simpler Times.

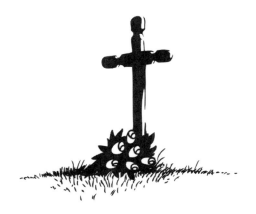

A VISIT WITH
MAMA AND GRANDMA

It is a tradition in South Georgia to periodically visit the burial plots of relatives who have passed on and make sure that the grounds are being kept, and to place some flowers at the gravesite. With Mother's Day coming up, Millard and Pedro decided to visit Mama's and Grandma's resting places and take some flowers.

Mama loved daisies. When Pedro was a little boy, he'd bring flowers to Mama and say, "Flowers for Mama, here's you a bouquet," and she'd hold him close. They weren't fancy and he'd picked 'em himself, but over the years they became Mama's favorite bouquet.

Pedro picked up Millard early one Sunday morning and went over to Mama's cemetery, which was located next to Colquitt Regional Medical Center on the south side of Moultrie. Pedro didn't know why the hospital and the cemetery were located next to each other. Upon arrival Pedro started walking slowly over to where Mama was resting and looked down. As Pedro stood there he realized how much he missed Mama. He recalled one time when the well went dry, he heard Mama say, "You don't miss the water until it's gone," and now, here on Mother's Day, Pedro knew exactly what she meant. Pedro then bent over and placed the flowers and once again said, "Flowers for Mama. Here's your favorite bouquet."

Without speaking a word, Millard and Pedro then left to go have a little talk with Grandma. She had been laid to rest next to Grandpa Williams at Big Creek Cemetery, south of Coolidge, Georgia. While traveling south on Highway 319, Pedro said to Millard, "We have a lot of relatives without problems, troubles, or worries, and all of 'em are equal. Most of 'em are resting at Hopewell Cemetery." Millard then said, "When you think you have a lot of problems and troubles, you need to think about that."

Upon arrival at Big Creek, they started walking toward Grandma's plot. They passed by one tombstone that said, "Devoted Family Man." The epitaph was either lying or the wrong person was in the hole. They then got over to Grandma's site and realized she still influenced their lives long after she had been gone. She had been a major character in their lives. At that moment Pedro remembered the words of poet Hugh Robert Orr:

> *They are not dead who live*
> *In lives they leave behind*
> *In those whom they have blessed*
> *They live a life again*
> *And shall live through the years.*

Upon standing over Grandma's grave, peacefulness set in and it seemed to help Pedro and Millard more than it helped Grandma. Pedro remembered that Grandma turned to family, a higher power, and to humor. She poked fun at herself and at things beyond her control. She said not to make a joke out of life, but a sense of humor would help us to tolerate the unpleasant and cope with the unexpected and it would add balance to the tightrope of life. As he stood there Pedro felt that he could almost hear Grandma still asking if he had on a clean change of underwear.

As Millard and Pedro continued to stand there, Pedro said, "Grandma, I made it. I'm a real doctor." He didn't have the heart to tell her that he was a radiologist. He just continued and said, "Grandma, I can now write prescriptions." Pedro silently thanked Grandma for inspiring, guiding, and prodding him to get his education.

By now the sun started goin' down and Millard and Pedro looked down at Grandmama's grave and began singing, "In the sweet by and by, we shall meet on that beautiful shore." Pedro took the low part and Millard took the high part. When it was all finished, Millard turned to Pedro and asked, "When I reach my journey's end, will you come on Father's Day and sing a song for me?" Pedro stood there lookin' directly at Millard with a lump in his throat unable to answer, but Millard already knew the answer and the sun finished goin' down.

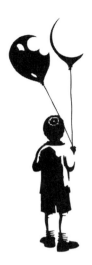

MOVIN' MADE EASIER

Frequent moves were not unusual for farm families back in the 1940s. There was always hope of a better year, a better home, better shoes, and a better crop.

In the mid-1940s Dad and the family, including Pedro, upped and moved to the north end of Colquitt County, but we still considered ourselves Southerners. This house had some indoor plumbing. It was amazing how that worked and the world was sure getting smarter. However, this place needed a whole lot of attention to make it look halfway decent and we upped and took it on ourselves to do that.

Dad had noticed that with this move, Pedro was getting down in the dumps. He asked Dillard to take Pedro fishing to get Pedro's mind on other things. Dillard and I then high-tailed it to Reedy Creek to do some jug fishing. The fish were biting so good we had to hide behind the tree to bait our hooks. We filled a No. 3 washtub plum full of fish. Dillard at the end of the day decided to drop by and give his brother Willard a mess of fish. After Dillard and I left Willard's and headed home to Millard's, Willard strung up his fish and had his picture taken. The next day Willard's picture came out in the *Moultrie Observer* holding the fish Dillard and I caught. The *Observer* had asked Willard in an interview where the fish were biting and he pointed to his upper lip and said, "Right here."

One time we were feelin' down and out and Dad recognized this. He scraped together some money, headed into town, and picked up a basket of apples, hopin' we'd all perk up. We thought Christmas had come early and that we were richer than we were. Pedro reached for one of them apples and bit into it faster than a rooster after a Junebug. Dad quickly said, "Pedro, be careful and look out for them worms." Pedro responded, "When I eat my apples, them worms have to look after themselves."

Even though times were sometimes tough, we kept our hopes up and for a long time Pedro kept hopin' for a bicycle. He was willing to give up his Easter outfit if only he could get that bike. Pedro thought he might be gettin' closer when he overheard Mama and Daddy talkin'. Dad told Mama that Pedro had been askin', beggin', and prayin' for a bike for a mighty long time and he asked Mama if she thought a bicycle might improve Pedro's behavior. Mama thought and said, "No, but it might spread it over a wider area."

We finally got settled in with this new move and the nearest neighbor was a long way off. During the summers we had to learn to occupy ourselves. I learned early not to complain of being bored or Dad would make me sweep the yard, wash the porch, dip the dog, haul some water, tote some wood, and weed the fields.

There was another share-cropper family down the road about one and a half miles and they had a boy about my age. I became close to him, played with him, picked cotton with him, and he taught me to ham-bone and I taught him to buck dance. He was black and he was my friend.

One day Dillard picked up a couple of balloons downtown — one was for me and one was for my friend. One balloon was black and one was white. This was a new type of balloon and would rise and had something inside called helium. My friend was excited and I was excited. In the excitement I let go of my balloon and it started rising higher and higher until it disappeared. My balloon had risen into the clouds. My friend looked at Uncle Dillard and asked, "Will my balloon rise as high as that white balloon?" Dillard replied, "It's not the color of the balloon that makes it rise, it's the stuff inside." I believed my friend had the right stuff inside. I wished I could find him now. I don't know where he has disappeared to but I'm sure he has risen above the clouds.

Repeated moving was hard on us kids. But concerned relatives and the warm reception from new good friends made it easier. Most of these relatives and friends have gone off in different directions and some already have passed on. They now are becoming the memories from which I draw strength when I reflect back on Simpler Times.

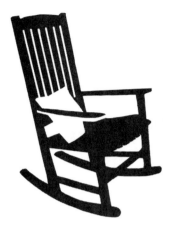

Family Reunions

Family reunions were a way of life in South Georgia, and the family reunion was coming up so I called home early in the morning to check on the situation. Grandma answered the phone. I said, "Grandma, I hope I didn't wake you up." She replied, "That's OK, I had to git up and answer the phone."

She told me that the reunion that year was at the Agricultural Building behind the Moultrie jail. Relatives were coming from Rome, Athens, Vienna, Cairo, Berlin, Boston, and lots of other places all over Georgia. Most of y'all probably didn't realize that Boston, Georgia, is the world's third-largest Boston. There were about eight-hundred people coming this year as usual, but it always seemed to be a different eight-hundred.

On the way to the reunion I passed by the ole homeplace and remembered Dad leaving Moultrie for the first time in 1944 to go way off across the water to fight in a war. He was scared. Mama was scared. She was alone with me and Mary Alice. Uncle Sam sent us a hundred dollars a month. Mama couldn't drive but it didn't matter 'cause we didn't have a car. The ice truck would come on Thursday and the rolling store would come on Tuesday. The rolling store was a truck that sold groceries, kerosene, etc. One day Mama was down to her last five dollars and I wanted some penny cookies. She allowed me to wait for the rolling store with the five dollars. Upon arrival I purchased five-hundred cookies and the rolling store pulled off. Mama started crying and then I started crying. We ate penny cookies for the next two weeks. I was always grateful to Mama after that for allowing me to live.

Finally, I arrived at the reunion and the first people I saw were Aunt Lourene and Uncle Ed. Uncle Ed was another one of Mama's half-brothers. We all hugged each other real tight and Aunt Lourene told me that Uncle Ed was doing real good. She said that he's now working with five-hundred people under him. I was real proud of the status he had now achieved even though he hadn't finished grammar school. She then said he was cutting grass at the Hopewell Cemetery.

I started wandering around and J.D. O'Kelly, one of my cousins, came up to me and showed me his sore finger. He wanted some medicine. I told him I was a radiologist. Later I heard him telling Willie that he thought Pedro had become a doctor, but come to find out Pedro's a radio man.

I continued mixin' and minglin' and bumped into Reuben, Daddy's sister's boy, who was a real doctor. He was practicing Ob-Gyn in Athens with his two brothers. He said, "Pedro, I worked real hard to get away from all of this. Now I have a place on half an acre in the suburbs and take call every third night. I now miss the Simpler Times and if only I could win the lottery I would come back and farm until the money ran out."

Later I went over to stand next to Grandma when one of the ladies walked by in a mini-skirt. Grandma turned to me and said, "Lordy mercy, Pedro. When I was a kid our skirts covered our in-steps. Her skirt doesn't even cover her step-ins."

Grandma was sitting in a rocker with a cushion. I noticed that bunches of people — five generations — were coming by and hugging her neck. She was the one who had brought all of us together. There were people from all walks of life including a lot of farmers, factory workers, builders, a few doctors, school teachers, road workers, and a grass cutter. There were old and young, people in suits, and people in overalls, those who were shy and others who made up for it. Yet, here we were — all gathered together once again with a similar upbringin' and raisin', but different, and still feeling a closeness. We were all brought back together to share moments and memories and to give our love to Grandma, the gentle lady with a wit who touched and influenced all our lives.

It started getting late and Grandma was getting tired. She told me she'd had all the fun she could stand and asked me to drive her home. On the way home, she looked over at me and said, "Pedro, you're big in my eyes and I love you." I said, "Grandma, you're big too and I love you." We didn't say another word the rest of the way home.

Then I started thinking that these big family reunions may become a thing of the past with everybody getting scattered ever' which way. The cousins had begun to quit farming and some left the county.

I knew the reunions wouldn't be the same when Grandma died, and they weren't.

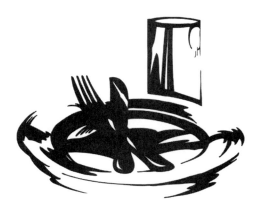

SUPPERTIME

Eatin' was simple in Simpler Times. It was simple 'cause you'd eat what they put in front of you. You did it for your health. If you didn't, Mama and Daddy would half-kill ya and Pedro learned early that complaining about your food was not good for ya.

Pedro also learned early about table manners. Mama told him not to chew with his mouth open, not to smack at the table, and not to put his elbows on the table. One time, Mama told Pedro to stop scratching his nose with his fork. Pedro responded by asking if it were more proper to use his spoon.

When we wanted food passed our way at the table, Pedro would say "thankee" for some taters and "thankee" for some cornbread. Mama said that we should be thankful because some people were starving and we should be thankful we weren't that poor. Sometimes Mama would take some leftovers to the poor family down the road. She said we owed it to them. They had lost their daddy in the war so we could have freedom to say what we wanted to and so us Baptists could practice our religion and make others do the same. Mama said us Baptists were like fish and would spoil if we stayed out of the water too long. Daddy said that if you're in deep water you needed to keep your mouth shut.

Meals represented a time for Mama and Daddy and us kids to sit down together with our heads bowed, and Dad would say the blessing. He was a simple man who tried to make a livin' diggin' in the soil but when he spoke, even a child could understand. There was food for the body and thoughts for the soul. He tried to teach us about sacrificing and sharing and about doing your part. He kept talkin' about gettin' your education and about being good to your neighbor. Dad once said that whatever you think about yourself is going to determine your future.

Conversation would often continue around the table and Grandma would join in. Pedro don't remember how old Grandma was but we had her for a long time. Grandma told us that ever' shut eye ain't sleepin' and ever' goodbye don't mean they're gone. We'd discuss the problems of the world and Mama said that the No. 1 problem was apathy. Grandma said that she didn't know what the word meant, but who cared?

Eatin' now is different in these so-called modern times. It has become difficult for many family members to join each other at suppertime and our eatin' habits have changed. Recently Dr. Zimmerman advised me that I needed to eat some tofu for protein and oat bran for fiber. Pedro had never heard of tofu. He never planted any or harvested any. I found some tofu at the New Leaf Market and it looked like low-cal fat-back. We used fat-back for seasoning of beans, greens, mustard, and collards and it was a staple item for cookin'. Prob'ly if we substituted tofu for fat-back it would give Southerners a bad attitude.

The memories of eatin' and of suppertime came back to me as I pondered over the years that have passed. Simpler Times has represented a way of life that is disappearing from the American scene. Some of the fondest memories of my childhood were woven around suppertime. If only I could go back to that old country place with ever'body joining together and once again hear Mama say, "Pedro, come on in. It's suppertime."

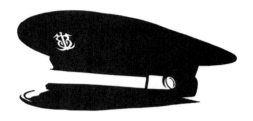

The Meaning
of Simpler Times

We spend the first half of our lives trying to git away from it and the last half trying to git back to it. Some folks move to the city so they can make enough money to move back to the country. It just seems that the grass always looks greener around the other fella's outhouse.

Often my thoughts drift back to Simper Times of childhood where I played around Mama's knee and heard her sing "Rock of Ages." Mama would remind us that ever' tub had to set on its own bottom and each person had to answer for themselves. Mama had a fear that us kids would grow up and hang around pool halls or grow up to be a Catholic. Mama would be happy to know that Pedro did neither. The closest he ever came to a Catholic was when he married one.

Mama always wanted us to do right and follow the Golden Rule. One time two brothers, R.T. and J.T., from down the road were fightin'. Mama hollored out, "Stop that. It's a downright dirty dog-rotten shame y'all got to act like that." She then asked, "Hadn't you boys ever heard of the Golden Rule?" R.T. hollored back and said, "Yes, ma'am, but J.T. didst unto me first."

Mama always talked as Pedro sat on the floor by her side. She pointed out that even though we were broke, we weren't poor and we had our kinfolks. They lived down the road and occasionally up the road, but not very far. They shared your joys, your hurts, and your beliefs. They helped look after you and they knew what you weren't supposed to be doing. They knew your dog's name and your dog's best friend.

When Pedro thinks back to his childhood, it seems that life wudn't complicated. It was simple for him 'cause Mama and Daddy gave him security, took care of him, and loved him. However, those times were not simple for them. They struggled to make ends meet, to provide for the kids, and to meet their obligations. It also was not simple 'cause Millard and Willard had to go off to fight in a world war. Pedro still felt secure 'cause he knew Millard and Willard were over there protecting him and Mama and the rest of the Country. Grandma spent her time on her knees asking God to bring her babies home safely. They did come home safely in their uniforms proud as a peacock and Grandma celebrated by once again falling on her knees and giving thanks. The rest of us stood there unable to speak with tears in our eyes waiting for our hug. Upon his return, the *Moultrie Observer* interviewed Millard and told him that it was wonderful that he would go over there across the water to die for his Country. He pointed out that wudn't quite true. He said, "I went over there to make some other fella' die for his Country."

Our parents always wanted us to have it better than them. They did not want us to forget our upbringing and where we came from. They had been through two world wars and a depression and survived. They just wanted life simple for us.

All of this may mean that Simpler Times means looking back to the past and to our childhood when we didn't have obligations and responsibilities, but did have unconditional love. Maybe we are building our own children's special moments and one day they may look back and say, "Back in Simpler Times ... ."

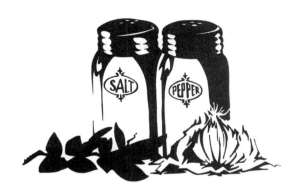

RECIPES
BONDS OF MEMORIES AND FOOD

The recipes in *More Simpler Times* are from Pedro's kinfolks and neighbors from his earlier years in South Georgia. Many of these kinfolks are no longer with us, but they continue to live on in Pedro's mind through his memories and their recipes. Specials memories were stored up and passed on around the supper table.

A lot of these recipes were handed down through many generations by word of mouth and with directions saying "a pinch of this" and "a dab of that." It is hoped that some of Pedro's memories and some of his relatives' recipes will be passed on and become part of his descendents' memories and bring joy to their hearts. It is also hoped that his folks will continue to get together for eatin', fellowship, and makin' new memories.

BEVERAGES

Apple Cider
Janice Harrell, Tallahassee, Florida

½ gallon apple cider
3 cinnamon sticks

½ cup sugar
¼ teaspoon ground cloves

Mix ingredients and simmer 30 minutes. May be served hot or iced.

Bridal Shower Pink Punch
Patricia Baker Williams, Tallahassee, Florida (wife of Pedro Williams)

1 package (3 ounces) strawberry Jell-O
1 package strawberry Kool-Aid
1 can (46 ounces) pineapple juice
2 pints lime sherbet

1 cup boiling water
2 quarts water
1 bottle (10 ounces) 7-Up
2½ cups sugar

Dissolve Jell-O in boiling water. Dissolve Kool-Aid in cold water. Add sugar and stir well. Add pineapple juice and Jell-O to Kool-Aid. Refrigerate. Add 7-Up and sherbet just before serving.

Lemonade
The festivity of Revival, of almost any picnic, or of a hot afternoon at home was heightened when a stone crock of tangy lemonade was brought out with a big, free-form piece of ice and thin slices of lemon floating on it. It would be ladled out into tall glasses and the cool

drink always fitted the occasion, whether it was chatting with friends under the shady oaks at Revival or relaxing at home after a hot morning of work in the fields. Often we would stir up a quick cake to serve with lemonade.

½ gallon well water
1½ cups freshly squeezed lemon juice
1 lemon, sliced into thin slices

2 cups sugar
ice
fresh mint (optional)

Dissolve the sugar in the well water (if you don't have a well, use bottled water). Add the lemon juice, a solid piece of ice, and lemon slices. This can be put into a stone crock or a glass bucket and decorated with mint, if desired. Makes 10 glasses.

Valentine's Day Sweetheart Punch
Mrs. Ella Wiard, Moultrie, Georgia

2 bottles (28 ounces each) cherry carbonated beverage (chilled)
1 jar (18 ounces) red maraschino cherries, drained
1 can (18 ounces) pineapple juice (chilled)
2 cans (13¼ ounces each) pineapple chunks, undrained
ice cubes

Combine ingredients in large punch bowl. Makes 25 ½-cup servings.

Party Punch

2 large cans pineapple juice
2 large cans orange juice
½ bottle real lemon juice

5 cups water
5 cups sugar
1 large bottle ginger ale

Mix all ingredients in large punch bowl and chill.

Old-Fashioned Lemonade
Patricia Baker Williams

1¼ cups fresh lemon juice
¾ cup sugar

4½ cups cold water
lemon slices

Combine lemon juice and sugar in a large pitcher; stir until sugar dissolves. Add water and lemon slices, stir well and chill. Serve over ice with lemon slices.

Dillon's Baptism Reception Punch
Patricia Baker Williams

This delicious springtime punch was served at the Baptism reception for Dillon Andrews on April 9, 1994.

1 can (12 ounces) frozen orange juice
1 can (6 ounces) frozen lemonade
1 can (6 ounces) frozen limeade
2 cans (46 ounces each) pineapple juice

6 cups water
2 2-liter bottles Sprite
lemon slices
strawberry slices

Use a decorative ring pan to make an ice-ring with one bottle of Sprite and the lemon and strawberry slices. Freeze. (Make several hours ahead.) Combine all juices with water and chill. When ready to serve, add chilled bottle of Sprite to the mix. Add frozen fruit ring to punch bowl. Serves about 27 guests.

BREADS

Crackling Bread
Mrs. Henry W. Lix

The skins and residue left from the renderings of pork fat at hogkilling time make cracklings. Ask a Southerner whose memory goes back far enough about crackling bread crumbled up in buttermilk – and watch his eyes light up!

2 cups cornmeal	½ teaspoon salt
1 teaspoon baking powder	⅔ cup cracklings

Sift into a bowl the cornmeal, baking powder, and salt. Pour into this enough boiling water to make a stiff batter. Add cracklings. Mold into oval shapes (pones) and bake in 425-degree oven until light golden brown. Serve with tall glass of very cold buttermilk, and instructions that hot crackling bread is to be broken up into the milk and eaten with iced teaspoons.

Corn Dumplings
Elois Gay Matthews

2 cups sifted corn meal	1 teaspoon baking powder
2 tablespoons butter	hot water
2 teaspoons salt	

Sift meal, salt, and baking powder together. Add melted butter to this and spoon-stir in enough hot water to make a dough. Form with hands into small balls. Drop these into boiling broth from pork or liquor from turnip greens. Simmer in covered pot about 30 minutes.

Sweet Potato Muffins
Judy Williams West (daughter of James Willard Williams)

1½ cups butter
1¼ cups sugar
2 eggs
¾ can of sweet mashed potatoes
1½ cups all purpose flour
2 teaspoons baking powder

1 cup milk
¼ cup chopped pecans
½ cup raisins
¼ teaspoon nutmeg
¼ teaspoon salt
1 teaspoon cinnamon

Cream butter and sugar, add eggs. Mix well. Blend in sweet potatoes. Sift in dry ingredients. Add alternately with milk. Fold in nuts and raisins. Put in greased muffin tins. Bake at 400 degrees for 25 minutes.

Sweat's Corn Fritters
Hugh Sweat

1 can (12 ounces) whole kernel corn
1 egg
½ cup Bisquick

½ teaspoon sugar
dash salt and pepper

Drain corn and mix with other ingredients. Deep fry in hot fat. Good with honey or syrup and fried white meat.

Hoe Cakes
Mrs. Henry W. Lix

Workers in the cotton fields first cooked this bread on their hoes over little campfires. It is also called "corn dodger."

4 cups cornmeal
1 teaspoon salt

boiling water
1 tablespoon bacon drippings

Scald cornmeal with enough boiling water to make a stiff dough. Add bacon drippings and salt. Shape into oval pones one handful of dough at a time, leaving the prints of the fingers across the top. Bake in greased baking pans at 425 degrees until light brown on one side. Turn and brown on the other side. This may also be cooked on top of the stove in a heavy iron skillet, turning them once to brown.

Hush Puppies

2 cups corn meal   1½ cups sweet milk
2 teaspoons baking powder   ½ cup water
1 large onion chopped fine   1 teaspoon salt

Sift dry ingredients together and add milk and water. Stir in chopped onion. Add more milk as may be necessary to form workable dough. Mold pieces of dough into pones (about 5" by 3" by ¾"). Fry in deep hot fat or oil until browned.

Corn Bread Dressing
Judy Williams West

2 cups cornmeal   1 teaspoon salt
½ cup shortening   2 eggs
1 teaspoon soda   2 cups buttermilk

Mix ingredients and bake at 425 degrees for about 20 minutes. Take cornbread and toasted bread and crumble up in large mixing bowl. Moisten with chicken broth. Add melted butter, onions, eggs, and chopped chicken. Salt and pepper to taste. Bake at 350 degrees for about 30 minutes or until onions are done. Reserve giblets for gravy. Boil about 3 eggs and take gizzard and liver and neck, chop this meat up fine. Take 1 ½ cups dressing and broth from chicken and cook on top of stove on medium heat until onions are done. Delicious!

Ginger Bread (Recipe over 100 years old)
Eudora O'Kelley

½ cup sugar
2 cups plain flour
½ teaspoon ginger
½ cup buttermilk
1 cup molasses (not syrup)

nuts and raisins to taste
½ cup shortening
½ teaspoon soda
½ teaspoon cinnamon

Mix sugar, shortening, and molasses until creamy. Mix in dry ingredients, then add buttermilk. Stir in nuts and raisins. Bake in large greased and floured pan for about 1 hour at 350 degrees.

Southern Cracklin' Cornbread
Eudora O'Kelley

4 cups cornmeal
1½ teaspoons salt
4 cups buttermilk
1 cup cracklings

2 teaspoons soda
4 eggs, beaten
⅓ cup bacon drippings

Combine cornmeal, soda, and salt. Stir in eggs and buttermilk. Heat bacon drippings in a 13" by 9" by 2" baking pan until very hot. Add drippings and cracklings to batter and mix well. Pour batter into hot pan. Bake at 450 degrees for about 25 minutes or until bread is golden. Cut into squares.

Banana Bread
Ophelia Williams Phillips (aunt of Pedro Williams)

1 cup flour
2 cups granulated sugar
3 large bananas, mashed

3 large eggs
1 cup salad oil
1 cup chopped pecans

Combine dry ingredients in mixing bowl. Add eggs and salad oil. Add bananas and nuts. Blend well. Bake at 350 degrees for 50 to 55 minutes in a loaf pan.

Old Fashioned Gingerbread
Mrs. Pat Edwards (aunt of Pedro Williams)

1 cup sugar	2 cups molasses
3 eggs	1 cup butter
3½ cups flour	1 cup sour milk
1 teaspoon ginger	½ teaspoon salt

Mix sugar and butter well. Add eggs one at a time, and then add sour milk and molasses (or any good South Georgia syrup) alternately with flour sifted with soda, salt, and ginger. Bake in a greased pan for about 40 minutes at 350 degrees.

Biscuits
Beverly Plymel

2 cups self-rising flour	¾ cup milk
½ cup solid shortening	

Preheat oven to 450 degrees. Lightly spoon flour into measuring cup and level off (do not pack flour). Cut shortening into flour until mixture resembles coarse meal. Add milk all at once and stir with a fork until a soft dough forms. Turn dough onto a lightly floured surface, sprinkle with flour and knead gently until dough is no longer sticky. Pinch off small amounts of dough and roll into a biscuit in palm of hand. Place on a greased cookie sheet and bake 8 to 10 minutes or until golden brown.

Note: You may substitute buttermilk and ¼ teaspoon soda for sweet milk.

Salads and Relishes

Easy Jell-O Salad
Mrs. Evelyn O'Kelly, Moultrie, Georgia

1 package (3 ounces) strawberry Jell-O
1 carton cottage cheese
1 tub (8 ounces) Cool Whip topping
1 can (15 ½ ounces) fruit cocktail, drained

Dissolve Jell-O in Cool Whip topping. Add cottage cheese and fruit cocktail. You may add ½ cup coconut or ½ cup nuts, if desired. Chill and serve.

Cole Slaw
Mary Alice Williams (sister of Pedro Williams), Moultrie, Georgia

1 medium cabbage
1 medium onion
3 carrots
1 cup mayonnaise

¼ cup vinegar
½ cup sugar
salt and pepper to taste

Grate cabbage, onions, and carrots in blender; add salt and pepper. Drain water off good. Mix mayonnaise, vinegar, and sugar together. Pour over cabbage mixture.

Refrigerator Pickles
Mrs. Reba Giddens (daughter of Willie Williams)

7 cups cucumber, sliced
1 cup onion, sliced
2 cups sugar

1 cup vinegar
1 tablespoon celery salt
2 tablespoons salt

Mix together and pour over cucumbers and onions. Put in big-mouth jar and keep in refrigerator.

Fourteen Day Cucumber Pickles
Mrs. Eula May Williams

2 gallons cucumbers
1 pint salt
2½ quarts vinegar

1 gallon boiling water
4 quarts sugar
alum

Mix ingredients and let stand 7 days. Take out cucumbers. Add another gallon boiling water. Let set 24 hours. Take out of water again and add 1 more gallon boiling water and 3 heaping tablespoons alum. Let stand 24 hours. Pour off and then do the rest: 4 quarts sugar, 2½ quarts vinegar. Boil 5 minutes. Pour over cucumbers. Do this for 5 mornings. Then put back in churn to keep. You do not have to can. Let stay in churn until gone.

VEGETABLES AND SIDE DISHES

Buttermilk Onion Rings
Lenora Davis, Moultrie, Georgia

2 large onions
2 eggs, separated
1¼ cups buttermilk
1½ tablespoons salad oil

1½ cup all-purpose flour
1 teaspoon salt
1¼ teaspoons baking powder

Peel onions and slice ½ inch thick; separate into rings. Beat egg yolks, add buttermilk and oil and sifted dry ingredients. Beat egg whites until stiff; fold in buttermilk mixture. Dip onion rings in batter. Fry a few at a time in deep fat at about 375 degrees. Drain on paper towel and sprinkle with salt. These may be frozen. When ready to serve, place on baking sheet and heat at 450 degrees for 5 minutes.

Sweet Potato Pone
Linda W. Cannon, Concord, California (sister of Pedro Williams)

2½ cups grated raw potatoes
1 cup sugar
2 eggs beaten
1 tablespoon grated orange rind
1 teaspoon nutmeg

2 tablespoons butter
1 cup chopped nuts
¼ teaspoon cinnamon
¾ cups sweet milk

Blend all ingredients; place in a buttered casserole and top with butter. Bake at 350 degrees until golden brown, about 45 minutes. Yields 6 servings.

Fried Okra

Select small, tender pods. Boil until tender, drain, season with salt and pepper, roll in beaten egg, then in corn meal. Fry in deep, hot fat.

Corn Pudding
Annie Laura Montgomery

2 cans creamed corn
2 eggs (slightly beaten)
1 stick margarine (melted)

16 saltine crackers (crushed)
⅔ cup milk
16 Ritz crackers (crushed)

Melt half of margarine in a small pan. Then mix corn, eggs, the melted margarine, saltine crackers, and milk. Put in a buttered Pyrex dish or pan the size of the silver rectangle biscuit pan. Top with the Ritz crackers and remaining margarine. I always melt the other half stick of butter and add my crumbs, crushed Ritz crackers, and mix till crackers are well coated. Then use your hand and sprinkle this over the top to cover it better, and kindly pat the cracker down a little with your hand. Bake at 300 degrees for 1 hour.

Randy's Elephant Stew
Randy Baker, Troy, Illinois

1 elephant
brown gravy
4 rabbits, optional

salt and pepper to taste
200 pounds, vegetables of choice

Cut elephant into serving-size pieces. Get help from a friend with a chainsaw! Add vegetables, elephant, and gravy. Cover and cook over low heat for three weeks. This will only serve 2,000 twice. If you expect a larger crowd, add the rabbit, but keep in mind some people won't like finding hares in their stew.

Fried Tomatoes

5 medium-sized tomatoes of good shape
½ cup unseasoned bread crumbs
2 tablespoons fresh bacon fat, or butter
½ cup flour
½ teaspoon salt
½ cup soft brown sugar
¼ teaspoon pepper

Sift the flour, bread crumbs, salt, and pepper. Slice off the top or stem end of tomatoes to get a flat slice. Cut ¼" slices and press each one into the flour mixture, coating both sides. Place the floured slices on a sheet of wax paper for a few minutes before cooking. Heat a skillet; when it is hot put in the bacon fat or butter, tilting the skillet to distribute it around the pan. When the butter is foaming or the bacon fat is smoking, put in the tomato slices and cook on a medium-high burner to obtain a good, brown crust. Cook for 4 minutes each side, turn the tomatoes over when browned, and sprinkle the browned top with ½ teaspoon brown sugar. Remove from the skillet and serve hot.

Corn Bread Dressing
Jewell Williams, Moultrie, Georgia

6 cups crumbled cornbread
4 cups loaf bread crumbled
1 cup chopped celery
3 teaspoon baking powder
¾ cup finely chopped onions
1 stick butter or margarine

2 teaspoons salt
⅛ teaspoon pepper
1 teaspoon poultry seasoning
4 eggs beaten
2 cups broth or milk

Prepare bread for dressing. Cook onions and celery in butter until tender. Add to bread crumbs and seasonings. Stir in beaten eggs and enough broth or milk to make the dressing moist. Dressing should be very moist. For extra fluffiness, stir in 3 teaspoons baking powder just before the mixture is poured into pan. Bake at 450 degrees until brown.

Potato Balls
Ray Tucker Family

Bread crumbs, about ¾ loaf
4 pieces celery, finely chopped
½ medium onion, diced
2 sticks butter, melted
1½ cups milk

2 eggs
salt and pepper to taste
2 cups mashed potatoes
a little sage

In a large bowl break up breadcrumbs. Mix rest of ingredients together with breadcrumbs. Place in a buttered pan with ice cream scoop. Melt half a stick of butter and spoon over each ball. Bake at 375 degrees for 20 minutes.

CASSEROLES AND MAIN DISHES

Hamburger Pie
Vivian Rogers

1 medium onion chopped
2 tablespoons fat
1 pound ground beef
½ teaspoon salt
¼ teaspoon pepper
1 cup cooked English peas

1 cup canned tomatoes
½ cup catsup
¾ cups self-rising corn meal
¼ cup self-rising flour
1 cup milk

Brown onions in fat; add meat. Cook until meat loses pink color and add salt, pepper, peas, tomatoes, and catsup. Pour into casserole dish. Combine meal and flour and milk, then drop from tablespoon over pie. Bake in preheated oven at 340 degrees for 30 minutes.

Pot Likker Dumplings
Mrs. Henry W. Lix

This originated in Tennessee, then traveled to Alabama and Texas more than 100 years ago. My mother learned to make them from my grandmother.

You must have one large pot of turnip greens boiled with ham hocks. Start from scratch, with turnip greens fresh out of the patch and smoked hambone or ham hocks. Or use chopped turnip greens canned, simmered an hour with the ham, which should already be boiled tender. Mix 2 tablespoons minced onion (fresh, young ones with part of the green tops are best) into 1½ cups unsifted cornmeal. Season with ½ teaspoon salt and ¼ teaspoon black pepper. Stir in enough boiling pot liquor from the greens to make stiff dough. When slightly cooled, mix in one egg thoroughly. Take this by spoonfuls and shape into small patties about ½" thick. Lay them gently on top of the simmering greens. Cover and simmer 10 to 15 minutes or until done.

Grand Slam Casserole
Ms. Gay Sanders, Moultrie, Georgia

1 pound ground beef
½ cup sliced onion
1 tablespoon butter
1 cup hot water
1 cup diced carrots

1 cup diced potatoes
2 cup canned tomatoes
1 ½ cups English peas (frozen)
1 teaspoon salt
1 cup biscuits (rolled ½ inch thick)

Brown meat and onions in butter. Add water and place in 2½ quart casserole. Cover and bake at 350 degrees for 30 minutes. Add remaining vegetables and seasoning. Cover and continue baking until vegetables are tender. Remove from oven. Place biscuits on top and bake 12 to 15 minutes. Yields 6 servings.

Georgia Chili
Shelby Plymel Macey

1 pound ground beef
salt and pepper
1 onion, chopped
3 tablespoons chili powder
1 tablespoon shortening

2 cups tomato juice
2 stalks celery, diced
1 green pepper, diced
1 can (15 ounces) tomatoes
1 can (15 ounces) kidney beans

Season ground beef with salt and pepper and 1 tablespoon chili powder. Brown seasoned beef and onions in shortening. Add tomato juice, celery, green pepper, and remaining chili powder; simmer slowly for 45 minutes or until vegetables are tender. If mixture cooks down, add more tomato juice or water. Add tomatoes, simmer 15 minutes longer. Add kidney beans, simmer 15 minutes more. Yields 6 servings.

Note: To save time and get rid of all the grease, I brown my beef and onion in a plastic colander sitting in a pie plate in the microwave. Afterwards, I cook everything except the kidney beans all day in a slow cooker; I add the kidney beans the last 15-30 minutes.

Country Pot Roast
Beverly Plymel

1 boneless beef chuck roast (about three lbs)
1 large onion, quartered
6 tablespoons all-purpose flour, divided
1 celery rib, cut in pieces
6 tablespoons butter or margarine, divided
1 teaspoon salt
3 cups hot water
½ teaspoon pepper

Sprinkle the roast with 1 tablespoon of flour. In Dutch oven, brown the roast on all sides in half the butter. Add the water, onion, celery, salt, and pepper; bring to a boil. Reduce heat, cover and simmer for 2 hours, or until meat is tender. Remove meat to a serving platter and keep warm. Strain cooking juices and set aside. In the same Dutch oven, melt remaining butter and stir in remaining flour; cook and stir until bubbly. Add 2 cups of the cooking juices and blend until smooth. Cook and stir until thickened, add additional cooking juices until gravy has desired consistency.

Beef and Vegetable Dumplings
Mrs. Lucile O'Kelley

2½ pounds beef stew
1 package frozen mixed vegetables
2 tablespoons Stero beef seasoning

1 package dumplings
1 large onion

Cook beef in six cups of water till tender. Add vegetables and seasoning and onion. Cook for 20 minutes. Add dumplings and cook until dumplings are done.

Chicken Pot Pie
Rosa Mae Weeks Plymel

2 cups (or more) cooked chicken, cut up
1 medium onion, chopped
4 boiled eggs, diced
2 cans cream of chicken soup
2 cans (16 ounces) Veg-All, drained
1 cup chicken broth
1 can (16 ounces) English peas, drained
1 cup mayonnaise (optional)

Mix all ingredients together or layer ingredients, if desired. Pour mixture into baking dish.

Topping
1 cup mayonnaise
1 cup self-rising flour
1 cup sweet milk

Mix topping ingredients together and pour over pie. Bake at 350 to 375 degrees for 1½ hours. Will serve 12 or more.

Corn Meal Dumplings
Lenora Davis

2 cups self-rising corn meal
½ cup self-rising flour
1 large onion, chopped fine
½ teaspoon black pepper

2 tablespoons melted shortening
1 egg
¾ cups buttermilk

Mix all ingredients together, adding only enough buttermilk to make a stiff dough. With your hands, make patties 2" square and ½" thick. Drop into 4 cups boiling liquid from cooked ham bone or shoulder bone. Cook 10 minutes or until done. Serve with cured ham or shoulder meat and vegetables.

Brunswick Stew
Jackie Plymel Connell

2 cans (or 1 quart) tomatoes
1 can boned chicken, or 1 fresh chicken
1 can barbecue beef
1 medium onion, sautéed in butter
1 tablespoon Tabasco sauce

2 cans cream style corn
1 can barbecue pork
1 teaspoon salt
1 tablespoon black pepper

Combine all ingredients and heat thoroughly. Makes about 3 quarts.

MEATS

Barbecued Chicken
Ms. Annie Williams (grandma of Pedro Williams)

1 fryer	1½ teaspoons red pepper
2 teaspoons catsup	1 well-greased paper bag
2 teaspoons vinegar	2 teaspoons lemon juice
2 teaspoons butter	1 teaspoon prepared mustard
1 teaspoon paprika	2 teaspoons Worcestershire sauce
4 teaspoons water	1 teaspoon chili powder

Take the chicken that has been cut and prepared for frying and thaw enough to take apart. In a large bowl, dip chicken in above ingredients mixed together. Place in well-greased bag and place on pan to cook 1 hour in 350-degree oven.

Skillet BBQ Pork Chops
Stephanie Flagg Andrews, Tallahassee, Florida

4 large boneless pork chops
¼ cup barbecue sauce (more if desired)
¼ cup water

Place pork chops in appropriate size skillet so chops are close but not overlapping. Add water and cover. Simmer on low to medium heat until chops are cooked completely. Add barbecue sauce, making sure both sides of chops are coated. Cover again and simmer on low for 10 to 15 minutes, turning chops once. Serve.

Hint: Barbecue sauce gravy is great over rice as a side dish.

Baked Rabbit

During the hunting season, a variety of game was bagged. Rabbit was the most plentiful and it kept very well. Most games can be kept, once the insides are removed, for a long period of time without being treated. We always left it hanging in fur or feathers during the winter and there was always rabbit for Christmas. We cooked it various ways, according to its age and tenderness. Baked in the wood cook oven was one way we loved it. It was simple, rich, and fine flavored.

1 3- to 4-pound rabbit	1 to 2 tablespoons flour
1 tablespoon soft butter	salt and pepper
1 medium onion, sliced	½ teaspoon thyme
1 cup water	smoked shoulder or bacon, sliced

Wipe the rabbit with a damp cloth, place in a baking pan, rub butter over, and sprinkle with salt, pepper, thyme, and a light sifting of flour. Place 2 or 3 slices of smoked shoulder of pork or bacon over the rabbit, a sliced onion, and spill a cup of water over. Cover the pan and set into a 350-degree oven for an hour and a half, opening the oven and basting every 15 to 20 minutes. When cooked, carve the rabbit and place on a platter. Dress the rabbit if it is your own game; with a store-bought rabbit, that won't be necessary.

Mom's Fried Chicken (Mom's most requested dinner)
Sharon and Charlie Dailey

chicken, enough for your family	seasoning salt
flour	salt and pepper
cooking oil	

In a large brown grocery bag, add a cup or two of flour and a good bit of pepper. Add salt. Shake to mix. Salt and pepper chicken pieces and sprinkle with seasoning salt. Add chicken pieces to flour mixture and shake until coated. Let sit awhile so chicken can become flavored with seasoning. Heat cooking oil till ready for frying. Fry chicken approximately 15 minutes on each side.

Country Fried Chicken
Jeanne Hensley Campise, Fresno, California

4 to 6 chicken breasts	4 ounces swiss cheese, grated
2 teaspoons paprika	4 tablespoons flour
2 teaspoons butter	1½ teaspoons salt
¼ cup dry sherry	1 tablespoon oil
¾ cup light cream or milk	⅓ cup dry white wine
1 tablespoon lemon juice	1 teaspoon cornstarch

Take split and skinned chicken breasts and slightly pound with side of saucer. Combine flour, paprika, and 1 teaspoon salt in bag. Shake chicken breasts in flour mixture several pieces at a time. Heat butter and oil over medium heat in a large skillet and brown chicken. Add sherry and cook, covered, 30 minutes or until chicken is just done. Remove chicken from pan and keep warm. Combine cornstarch, cream or milk, and ½ teaspoon salt and stir into pan drippings. Cook over medium heat until slightly thickened, about 10 minutes. Add wine and lemon juice and heat through. Place chicken back in sauce and top with swiss cheese. Cover and keep over low heat until cheese melts.

Meat Loaf
Mary Fabian Brady Austin, Morganfield, Kentucky

This is as close to my mother's recipe, Opal Brady, as I can come. My husband, who never liked meatloaf, really eats this well. My children love it cold on a sandwich, if any survives to be eaten later.

1½ pounds ground beef	¼ teaspoon pepper
¾ cups oats, uncooked	1 cup catsup
¼ cups chopped onion	1 egg, beaten
1½ teaspoon salt	

Combine all ingredients thoroughly. Pack firmly into an ungreased 8¼" by 4½" by 2½" loaf pan. Bake at 350 degrees for 1 hour and 15 minutes. Drain liquid. Top with catsup and cook another 10 minutes. Let stand 5 minutes before slicing. Yields 8 servings.

Roast Stuffed Coon

After coon has been skinned, defatted and deglanded, wipe with damp cloth. Dust outside with baking soda, rubbing it into the meat. Rinse in 2 or 3 changes of cold water. Put into roasting pan and add the following: water to just cover, 2 chopped carrots, 2 chopped onions, 2 stalks chopped celery. Cover and simmer for 30 minutes. Remove and allow to cool, then rub inside and out with a mixture of 2 parts salt and 1 part pepper. To make dressing, mix the following:

2 quarts bread crumbs	1 beaten egg
1 teaspoon salt	1 chopped onion
¼ teaspoon pepper	1 sliced apple
1½ teaspoon poultry seasoning	1 cup milk or 1 cup broth

Stuff and skewer, add a little water, cover pan tightly, and roast at 350 degrees until tender. Baste often and brown, as with a turkey.

DESSERTS

Fresh Blackberry Cobbler

Blackberries were always a favorite with us. The berries grew abundantly in the woods and in the fields. We would go out early in the morning to pick them, gathering a quart or a gallon in a very short time. You need to look out for rattlesnakes and be prepared to scratch red bug bites. Everyone looked forward to a pie or a cobbler during the season. The cobbler was baked in a large, deep baking pan with a delicious crust made from home-rendered lard and baked to a golden brown, with syrupy juice spouting through the pierced top as the berries cooked. It was served warm with the delicious juice from the berries spooned over the top.

Pastry
2 cups sifted unbleached flour   ⅓ cup cold water
½ teaspoon salt   1 cup crushed cube sugar
½ cup lard   ¼ cup light cream

Filling
5 cups blackberries   ¾ cup granulated sugar
4 thin slices butter   2 teaspoons cornstarch

Sift the flour and the salt into a large mixing bowl. Blend in the lard with a pastry blender or your fingers. When it is well-blended and fine-grained, sprinkle all the water in at once and draw the dough together quickly, shaping it into a ball. Divide in half and let stand for a few minutes. After it has rested, roll out one piece and line the baking pan. Sprinkle 2 or 3 tablespoons of the crushed sugar over the dough, cover with wax paper, and set it into the refrigerator (or freezer) until you are ready to fill it, along with the other piece of dough. When you are ready to assemble the cobbler, remove the dough from the refrigerator and roll out the top crust. Remove the pastry-lined pan from the refrigerator and fill it with berries, distributing the pieces of butter and sprinkling over the ¾ cup granulated sugar mixed with cornstarch. Wet the rim of the dough in the pan and place the top pastry over, pressing down all around to seal and trimming away excess. With the handle of a dinner knife, make a decorative edge and then cut a few slits in the center to allow steam to escape. Brush the top with a thick brush of cream and sprinkle on the remaining crushed cube sugar. Place in a preheated 450-degree oven and when the door is shut, turn down to 425 degrees to bake for 45 minutes. Remove from the oven and set on a rack to cool a bit before serving.

Making Ice Cream on a Summer Afternoon

Ice cream making was another family affair. Many hands were welcome for turning the crank. It is always wise to make the custard early and set it to chill in the refrigerator.

Vanilla Custard Ice Cream

2 cups milk	¼ teaspoon salt
½ vanilla bean (open a bit)	1 tablespoon vanilla extract
4 egg yolks, beaten	1 quart heavy cream
1 cup sugar	1 1-gallon freezer
5 pounds rock salt	1 5-pound bag ice
1 cork for freezer top	8" by 8" by 2" baking pan

Pour the milk into a saucepan to scald. Add vanilla bean and have the burner medium high. The milk has reached a scald when tiny beads form around the edge of the milk. Never allow it to boil. Have at hand a bowl containing the beaten yolks with sugar and salt added. Remove vanilla bean and pour the milk slowly into the yolk mixture while stirring constantly. Pour the mixture into a clean saucepan and set over a medium-high burner, stirring continuously until the milk begins to heat. Lift the pan up and hold above the burner. Raise the flame a bit and stir until a definite coat covers the spoon, about 3 to 4 minutes. Set the pan into a bowl of cold water to halt cooking. Strain the custard into a bowl and cool. When cold, add vanilla and heavy cream. Stir well, cover, and set in refrigerator to chill. It is good to scald the freezer can, dasher, and cover, and set them to chill as well. Have ice crushed small enough to fit properly between can and bucket. Have the salt and bucket at hand. Stir the custard well. Put dasher in place and stir in custard. Fill three-quarters full. Attach the crank, lock, and turn very gently to see if it's on correctly. Fill with ice and salt – first a layer of ice, then a layer of salt, repeating until the bucket is filled to the top. Use 3 parts ice and 1 part salt, always being careful not to get any salt into the cream from the top of the can. Turn the can gently the first few turns, then turn as fast as you can, exchanging with someone else as you tire. The ice will be melting continuously as you turn. This is necessary to freeze the cream. Never let it reach the top of the can because it may get into the cream. Tilt can on the side with hole to draw off water. Refill with ice and salt.

As the cream begins to freeze it will become harder to turn. Continue to turn until it becomes almost impossible – about 25 to 30 minutes. Tilt the bucket to drain out water. Unlock crank and lift it off. Wipe off the top of the cream can in place while you lift out the dasher. With a long-handled spoon, scrape the cream from the dasher, lay the dasher on the platter or hand it to the children who usually are waiting to lick it. Dip the spoon into the cream and bring up the frozen part from the bottom by folding the top in. Do this folding motion 3 or 4 times. Smooth over and replace the cover. Place the cork in the opening of the cover and pack it again with salt and ice as you did before freezing. Cover with burlap bag or heavy cloth. Set in bottom of the refrigerator or a cool place for at least 2 to 3 hours before using. Makes about 2 quarts.

Pecan Pie

3 eggs
1 cup sugar
½ cup Karo syrup

¼ cup melted margarine
1 cup pecans, chopped
1 pie crust

Turn oven to 375 degrees. Beat eggs slightly in a 2-quart bowl. Stir in sugar, corn syrup, and melted butter. Mix well after each. Stir in pecans. Pour into unbaked pie shell. Bake 35 to 40 minutes or until filling is slightly firm.

Ritz Cracker Pie

2 cups water
1½ cups sugar
pie shell
butter

2 teaspoons cream of tartar
20 Ritz crackers
cinnamon

Bring to a hard boil. Then drop in 20 Ritz crackers. Boil 2 or 3 minutes. **Do not stir.** Let cool for 15 minutes. Pour into unbaked pie shell. Sprinkle with cinnamon and dot with butter generously. Put on top crust. Bake 10 minutes at 400 degrees, then turn down oven to 375 degrees and bake 20 minutes.

Fudge Filled Peanut Butter Bars
Kathryn C. Goble, Barney, Georgia (cousin of Pedro Williams)

1 package yellow cake mix
1 cup peanut butter

½ cup butter or margarine, melted
2 eggs

In large mixing bowl, combine dry cake mix, peanut butter, butter, and eggs; stir until dough holds together. Press ⅔ of dough into bottom of ungreased jelly roll pan or 13" by 9" baking pan. Reserve remaining dough for topping. Prepare filling according to directions below and spread over dough in pan. Crumble reserved dough over filling, press lightly into filling. Bake at 350 degrees for 20 to 25 minutes until lightly browned. Cool and cut into bars.

Filling
1 cup flaked coconut
2 tablespoons margarine
½ teaspoon salt
15 ounces condensed milk

2 cups semi-sweet chocolate pieces
1 cup chopped nuts
2 teaspoons vanilla

In heavy sauce pan, combine chocolate, milk, butter, and salt. Melt over low heat, stirring constantly until smooth. Remove from heat; add coconut, nuts and vanilla.

Apple Dumplings
The Late Pearlie Lairsey

2 cups water
1½ cups sugar
¼ teaspoon cinnamon
½ teaspoon nutmeg
8 drops red food coloring
½ cup butter

1 cup sifted flour
2 teaspoons baking powder
1 teaspoon salt
¾ cup shortening
½ cup milk
6 apples, peeled and cored

Mix first 5 ingredients and cook 5 minutes to make basting mixture. Remove from heat and add butter. In separate bowl, sift dry ingredients and cut shortening to make coarse meal. Add milk and stir until dry ingredients are moistened. Roll out dough to make 6 squares. Place an apple on each and sprinkle with sugar, cinnamon, and nutmeg. Brush dough with butter and bring corners to center to form jacket (tuck in apple cavity). Place apple dumplings in basting mixture and baste dumplings. Bake at 375 degrees for 35 to 40 minutes, basting often while cooking. Serve with cream.

Sweet Potato Balls
The Late Mary Savannah Williams (mama of Pedro Williams)

crushed cornflakes
¼ cup pineapple juice

2 cups hot mashed sweet potatoes

Combine cooked potatoes and juice and beat until smooth. Then form into balls the size of small eggs. Roll these in crushed cornflakes. Place in a buttered shallow 2-quart baking dish and bake at 325 degrees for 25 minutes.

Lemon Cheese Cake
Charles D. "Pedro" Williams, MD, Tallahassee, Florida

1 cup butter	3 cups sifted cake flour
2 cups sugar	¾ cup milk
1 tablespoon baking powder	6 egg whites beaten stiff

Cream butter and sugar with mixer, beat until light and fluffy. Add sifted dry ingredients alternating with milk; fold in egg whites. Pour into 3 greased, round 8" layer pans. Bake at 350 degrees for 25 to 30 minutes.

Filling

½ cup butter	6 egg yolks
1 cup sugar	2 lemons

Use juice from lemons and grate rind; combine all ingredients in iron skillet and cook over low heat, stirring constantly until thick. Cool, then place between layers and on top of cake.

Banana Pudding
Lenora Davis, Moultrie, Georgia

1 package (6 ounces) vanilla pudding	2½ cups milk
1 box (12 ounces) vanilla wafers	6 ounces sour cream
12 ounces whipped topping	4 large bananas

Mix vanilla pudding with milk according to directions on box. Add sour cream and mix well. Fold whipped topping into mixture until well blended. Place a layer of vanilla wafers on bottom of large deep dish, then a layer of bananas, sliced. Cover bananas with half the pudding mix, repeat with the rest of bananas then rest of pudding mix. To dress it up, sprinkle vanilla wafer crumbs on top. Refrigerate until ready to serve. Serves 6 to 8.

Sweet Tater Stuff
Rosa Mae Weeks Plymel, Gail Weeks and Pearlie Lairsey
Autryville, Georgia

3 cups cooked, drained, mashed sweet potatoes
⅓ cup butter or margarine
2 eggs
1 teaspoon vanilla
1 cup sugar

Blend ingredients together well and pour in greased pan or dish, never more than 1" deep.

Topping

1 cup light brown sugar
⅓ cup flour

1 cup chopped pecans
⅓ cup margarine, softened

Cut flour, sugar, and margarine with 2 knives till coarse, add nuts and spread over potatoes. Bake at 350 degrees for 30 minutes. This can be frozen before or after baking.

Peanut Brittle
Edna Coombs, Tallahassee, Florida

2 cups sugar
1 cup light corn syrup
1 teaspoon butter or margarine
¾ teaspoon soda

½ teaspoon salt
1 cup water
2 cups unroasted Spanish peanuts

Combine sugar, corn syrup, and water in heavy boiler, then cook slowly until sugar dissolves. Cook to softball stage. Do not stir unless needed. Add peanuts and salt. Cook to hard crack stage, stirring constantly. Add butter and soda, stir to blend. Mixture will bubble. Pour onto buttered large platter or baking pan. Cool, then break into pieces. Make sure pan is buttered well or brittle will stick.

Poor Man's Cobbler
Bonnie S. Tolbert

This is my dad, Joe Beaven's favorite recipe. He was always the baker when Ruthie and I were growing up. Mother did the main part of the meal, but Daddy did the baking. He especially loved baking pies.

1 stick margarine
1 cup flour
1 cup sugar
1 cup milk

1 teaspoon baking powder
1 large can fruit
pinch salt

Put stick of margarine in 13" by 9" baking pan. Place in oven and pre-heat to 350 degrees. Mix together flour, sugar, milk, baking powder, and salt. Pour in pan with melted margarine. Spread can of fruit over batter in pan and bake for 45 minutes.

Mountain Dew Cake
Louise Driver Neely

Cake
1 box yellow cake mix
1 can (12 ounces) Mountain Dew
1 pkg. pineapple instant pudding

½ cup Crisco oil
4 eggs

Topping
1 can (12 ounces) crushed pineapple
1½ cups sugar

4 tablespoons flour

Mix cake ingredients and bake; make 3 layers. Boil topping ingredients for 5 minutes, or until clear and thick. Cool to lukewarm and spread over cake.

Ice Box Fruit Cake
The Late Sallie Lou P. Murphy (grandma of Pedro on his mama's side)

1 pound marshmallows
1 can (5 ounces) evaporated milk
1 pound Graham crackers
1 pound raisins

4 cups chopped nuts
12 ounces dates
1 jar Maraschino cherries

Melt marshmallows in milk on top of double boiler. Crush crackers. Mix cracker crumbs, nuts, raisins, and dates and add to marshmallow mixture. Then add cherries and mix well. Pour into a pan lined with wax paper and let set until firm. Refrigerate.

Christmas Fruitcake
Late September was a fine time to make the Christmas fruitcake. There were rainy days in September when outside work was curtailed and the cookstove was on, making the kitchen warm and cozy. The family was around and friends were dropping in – chopping fruit, grinding spices, and sampling homemade wine, trying to decide which one was best for the cake, and sipping a bit of whisky as well. Preparing the cake became a festive occasion, and almost as exciting as Christmas itself.

In selecting ingredients for the fruitcake, it is best to buy a few important items such as citron, seeded raisins, and candied peel in late December for the following Christmas. The freshest ingredients come into the market too late to make an aged cake. The special fruits can be kept perfectly well in a cooled, dry place (not in refrigerator) until it's time to make the cake. The same care should be taken with spices. Cinnamon from Ceylon is much more delicate and sweet than the other bark that is found today at most fancy food places.

Fruitcake is so special and lasts so long that only the best ingredients should be used in it. When Dad was in World War II in Belgium, Mama sent him a fruitcake for Christmas. The fruitcake followed him around the world during the war and never quite reached him. Six months after the war was over and Dad returned home, the fruitcake arrived back in Moultrie, Georgia. This was the best eatin' and best gatherin' and best joy we had in the 1940s. We figured it had aged enough.

2 cups (1 pound) butter	10 medium-sized eggs, well-beaten
2 cups granulated sugar	2 cups soft brown sugar

1 cup unsulphured molasses	1 cup sorghum molasses
1 cup grape jelly	1 cup blackberry wine

⅔ nutmeg, grated
1 teaspoon freshly ground cloves
2 teaspoons freshly ground allspice
2 teaspoons freshly ground mace
2 teaspoons freshly grated Ceylon cinnamon
2 tablespoons vanilla extract

8 cups sifted unbleached flour   4 teaspoons Royal baking powder

2 pounds seeded muscrat raisins (seed by hand preferably)
2 pounds seedless dark raisins
1 pound citron, sliced thin and cut into ½ inch pieces
1 pound currants
½ pound each candied orange and lemon peel (can be homemade)

2 cups rum or brandy

Cream the butter and sugars until light. Add beaten eggs and mix well while stirring in molasses, jelly, and wine. Stir in spices, vanilla, and flour with baking powder added. Add in the fruit bit by bit, stirring well after each addition. When well-mixed, spoon the batter into 2 10" tube pans, greased and lined on bottoms and sides with uncontaminated brown paper (makes about 17 pounds of batter for two large cakes). Fill three quarters full and set the pans in an odorless, cold place for 2 days. Then set the cake batter into a preheated oven that ranges between 250 degrees and 300 degrees for 4 hours. Remove from oven and cool in pans. When cold, remove from pans and leave cakes encased in paper wrapping; store in clean, dry tins or wooden boxes (any container other than plastic). Lace the cakes beginning in early December once a week with ½ cup rum or brandy. Lace for 4 weeks. Keep the containers covered.

Homemade Banana Pudding
Debbie Flagg, Miami, Florida

3½ tablespoons all-purpose flour
1 box (12 ounces) vanilla wafers
1⅓ cups sugar
¼ cup + 2 tablespoons sugar
3 eggs, separated, room temperature

6 medium bananas
3 cups milk
2 teaspoons vanilla
dash salt

Combine flour, 1⅓ cups sugar, and salt in a heavy saucepan. Beat egg yolks and combine with milk, mixing well, then stir into dry ingredients. Cook over medium heat, stirring constantly, until smooth and thickened. Remove from heat; stir in 1 teaspoon vanilla. Layer a third of the wafers in a 3-quart baking dish. Slice two bananas and layer over wafers. Pour ⅓ custard over bananas. Repeat layers twice. Beat egg whites until foamy. Gradually add remaining sugar a tablespoon at a time, beating until stiff peaks form. Add 1 teaspoon vanilla and beat until blended. Spread meringue over custard, sealing to edge of dish. Bake at 425 degrees for 10 to 12 minutes or until golden brown. Yields 8-10 servings.

Divinity
Jewell Williams

2½ cups sugar
½ cup light corn syrup
¼ teaspoon salt
½ cup water

1 teaspoon vanilla
2 egg whites
cinnamon candy (optional)

Combine, sugar, syrup, salt, and water in 2-pint saucepan. Cook on high until mixture reaches 260 degrees (hard ball stage) on candy thermometer; stir only until sugar dissolves. Remove from heat; cool for 3 to 4 minutes. Beat egg whites to stiff peaks. Gradually pour syrup over egg whites in a thin stream, beating at high speed on electric mixer. Add vanilla and beat until candy holds its shape and starts to lose its gloss. Quickly drop from teaspoon onto wax paper. Top with cinnamon candy if desired. Store in air-tight container. Yields 3 dozen.

Aunt Pat's Cherry Cream Cheese Tarts
Patricia Baker Williams

16 ounces cream cheese
1 package vanilla wafers
2 eggs
muffin papers

1 teaspoon vanilla
1 can cherry pie filling
¾ cup sugar

Beat cream cheese, eggs, sugar, and vanilla together with electric mixer until creamy. Place one vanilla wafer on bottom of each muffin paper. Fill muffin cups half full of mixture. Spoon a little pie filling over mixture. Bake at 375 degrees for approximately 15 minutes.

Sunday Syrup
Mrs. Leslie Williams

½ cup cocoa
1½ cups sweet milk

3 cup sugar
1 stick butter or margarine

Using heavy sauce pan, mix sugar and cocoa, then add milk. Bring to rolling boil. Add butter. Serve over hot biscuits, along with fried ham or sausage.

Pecan Pie
Linda W. Cannon (sister of Pedro Williams)

1 cup sugar
1 cup white Karo syrup
1 cup chopped pecans
¼ teaspoon salt

2 eggs, well beaten
¼ cup butter or margarine
1 unbaked 9" pastry shell

Cream butter and sugar. Add salt, eggs, syrup, and chopped nuts; mix well. Pour into pastry shell and bake at 300 degrees for 1 hour.

Watermelon Filled with Fruit and Dip
Diane and Mickey Andrews (Stephanie's in-laws)

Fruit
Watermelon
Grapes
Strawberries
Cantaloupe
Any other fruit of choice

Dip
8 ounces cream cheese
7 ounces marshmallow cream
¼ teaspoon almond extract
1 teaspoon vanilla
2-3 drops red food color

Blend dip ingredients with mixer until smooth. Hollow out watermelon. Remove seeds. Add cut-up watermelon and remaining fruit to the watermelon half, which is used as a serving bowl. Dip fruit into dip with toothpicks. Eat on the back porch so the juice can run down your elbows.

Sweet Potato Pie
Mary C. Beaver, Louisville, Kentucky

½ teaspoon cinnamon
3 large yams
2 cups sugar
2 tablespoons vanilla

3 large eggs
1 stick butter or margarine
½ tablespoon nutmeg

Scrub and boil yams, slip off skins. While still hot, place in electric mixer bowl with butter. Beat at high speed until smooth. Add eggs and sugar. Beat until consistency of cake batter. Season with cinnamon, nutmeg, and vanilla. Pour into unbaked pie shell. Bake at 350 degrees for 40 to 50 minutes or until toothpick inserted in center comes out clean. Can be frozen up to 6 months.

THIS AND THAT

Dishpan Dressing
The Late Mary Savannah Williams

4 cups self-rising corn meal
2 cups milk
4 large onions chopped

1 loaf toasted bread
16 eggs
salt and pepper

Mix corn meal, milk, onions and 4 eggs together to make cornbread and bake until brown. Let cool before using. Combine cornbread that has been crumbled, light bread, remaining dozen eggs, and salt and pepper to taste. Mix in broth of turkey or large hen that has been boiled. Mix together with potato masher and pour in dishpan. Needs to be soupy; if needed, add water. Don't forget to save some mixture for Giblet Gravy (see recipe below). Bake at 400 degrees until golden brown.

Giblet Gravy
The Late Mary Savannah Williams

liver
gizzard
neck
4 boiled eggs, chopped

salt and pepper
2 cups dressing mixture
½ cup cooked celery

Boil liver, gizzard, and neck; chop fine. Add to broth of giblets and stir in eggs, dressing mixture, and celery, and salt and pepper to taste. Cook together until mixture thickens.

5-Minute Homemade Barbecue Sauce
Mrs. Pat Edwards

5 ounces A-1 Steak Sauce
1¼ cups catsup
1 can (6 ounces) orange juice concentrate (or ¼ cup brown sugar)

Combine ingredients. Bring to a boil and simmer 5 minutes. Baste while barbecuing. Sauce is excellent on beef, chicken, spare ribs, or pork. May be stored in refrigerator for 2 to 3 weeks.

Country Skillet Milk Gravy
Mary Alice Williams

4 tablespoons meat drippings   2 cups milk
3 tablespoons self-rising flour   salt and pepper to taste

Spoon flour into drippings and blend over low heat until smooth; brown lightly. Gradually add milk while constantly stirring until thick. Season with salt and pepper.

Fig Preserves
Mary L. Smith

4 quarts fresh figs with stems   8 cups sugar
1 tablespoon soda   1 quart water
3 cups boiling water   1 lemon, thinly sliced

Place figs in large bowl; sprinkle with soda. Add 3 quarts boiling water, and soak 1 hour. Drain figs; rinse thoroughly in cold water. Combine sugar and 1 quart water in a large Dutch oven; bring to a boil, and cook 10 minutes. Add figs and lemon to syrup; cook until figs are clear and tender (about 1 hour), stirring occasionally. Spoon figs into hot sterilized jars; if necessary, continue cooking syrup until thick. Pour syrup over figs, leaving ⅛" head space. Run knife around edge of jars to remove air bubbles. Top with lids and screw metal bands tight. Process 10 minutes in boiling water bath. Yields 4 to 5 pints. The remaining syrup can be poured into a hot sterilized jar, sealed, processed, and used as topping for pancakes, toast, or ice cream.

Tomato Catsup
The Late Mary Savannah Williams

1 gallon ripe tomatoes	1 tablespoon ground mustard
1 quart vinegar	1 cup brown sugar
1 tablespoon salt	1 teaspoon ground cinnamon
1 tablespoon red pepper	½ teaspoon cloves
1 tablespoon black pepper	2 large onions

Boil 4 hours and run through a sieve. Heat catsup again until very hot. Seal in bottles.

Farmer's Breakfast
Patricia Baker Williams

6 slices bacon	salt and pepper to taste
½ cup green pepper, diced	½ cup cheese of choice, grated
¼ cup onion, diced	6 eggs, beaten well
3 large potatoes	

Fry bacon. Cut in small strips. Save 3 tablespoons of bacon grease in skillet and add green pepper and onion. Add boiled, peeled, and cubed potatoes to skillet and sprinkle with salt and pepper. Fry until golden brown, stirring often. Add bacon to potatoes and pour into 13" by 9" baking dish sprayed with PAM. Add eggs to potato mixture. Sprinkle cheese over eggs. Bake at 350 degrees for about 30 minutes.

Mamma Baker's Giblet Gravy
Patricia Baker Williams

This Giblet Gravy was always a family tradition at our house for
Thanksgiving and Christmas.

4 boiled eggs	corn starch for thickening
giblets from turkey	turkey neck
broth from turkey	

Fill large pot ¾ full of water. Add whole turkey neck and whole giblets. Simmer-boil for about 2 hours or until meat or turkey neck and
gizzard is very tender. Remove neck and giblets, let cool. Strip meat
from neck and cut in small pieces. Dice giblets into small pieces. Return cut-up meat to water they were cooked in and continue to simmer. Add finely chopped eggs. Pour off turkey broth from already
cooked turkey and add broth to gravy (about 3 cups). Let gravy cook
for a little while after eggs are added. Mix your favorite thickening
(Mom used corn starch) and add to gravy. Let cook a bit longer until
thickened. Delicious served with turkey and dressing.

Betti's Fluffy Pancakes
Betti Butler, Troy, Alabama

½ cup butter	½ cup flour
2 eggs	dash salt
½ cup milk	dash nutmeg

Heat oven to 425 degrees. Melt butter in 12" iron skillet or other appropriate baking pan in oven. Mix eggs, milk, flour, and seasonings in
blender. Pour mixture into hot skillet and bake 10 to 15 minutes until
puffy and golden brown. Top with powdered sugar, jams, hot apple
sauce, or other toppings that you enjoy. Serves 8.

Red-Eye Gravy

After frying a slice of country ham, drain off excess fat, add a little water to the drippings and about a tablespoon of strong coffee for color. Bring to a boil and serve with the ham.

Best Play Dough – Not for eating!
Betti Butler, Troy, Alabama

Children love this recipe. It is even better than store-bought because you can add water to it when it begins to dry out. I got this recipe from a friend of mine while living in Duluth, Georgia. My sister, Pat, and her children had come to visit us (my children were young then also). It was a rainy day and our children were getting restless so I called my friend who I knew had made this recipe for her children and asked her for it. Well, this recipe literally saved the day! Our children played with it for hours and had a wonderful time!

1 cup flour
1 cup water
4 teaspoons cream of tartar
1 cup salt
2 teaspoons cooking oil

Mix together and cook over medium heat until thick, stirring vigorously on the bottom of pan to prevent sticking. Turn out onto counter top and knead until soft and smooth. At this point you can divide it into parts and add a different color of food coloring to each part. Store in plastic bags in refrigerator when not in use. It can be stored at room temperature if preferred but will not last long as the oil turns rancid in time. Supply the children with rolling pins (empty vegetable cans work also) and cookie cutters.

By the way, they will also enjoy it much more if you sit down at the table and play with it with them – at least at first, anyway!

Recipe Notes

Recipe Notes

Recipe Index

more simpler times
Book Order Form

PRICE: $19.95 per book
SHIPPING: $ 3.00 per book

SHIP TO:

Name: _____

Address: _____

City: _____ State:_____ Zip:_____

Quantity:_____ x   Price: $_____   = Total: $_____

Quantity:_____ x   S&H: $_____   = Total: $_____

ORDER TOTAL: $_____

Make checks payable to Capital Medical Society Foundation. Please detach form and mail with payment to **1204 Miccosukee Road, Tallahassee, FL 32308.** Allow four weeks for delivery.